Working with older people and their families

edited by
Mike Nolan, Sue Davies and Gordon Grant

D1008957

Open University Press
Buckingham · Philadelphia

Open University Press
Celtic Court
22 Ballmoor
Buckingham
MK18 1XW

email: enquiries@openup.co.uk
world wide web: www.openup.co.uk

and
325 Chestnut Street
Philadelphia, PA 19106, USA

First Published 2001

Copyright © Editors and contributors, 2001

All rights reserved. Except for the quotation of short passages for the purpose of criticism and review, no part of this publication may be reproduced, stored in a retrieval system, or transmitted, in any form or by any means, electronic, mechanical, photocopying, recording or otherwise, without the prior written permission of the publisher or a licence from the Copyright Licensing Agency Limited. Details of such licences (for reprographic reproduction) may be obtained from the Copyright Licensing Agency Ltd of 90 Tottenham Court Road, London, W1P 0LP.

A catalogue record of this book is available from the British Library

ISBN   0 335 20560 7 (pb)   0 335 20561 5 (hb)

Library of Congress Cataloging-in-Publication Data
Working with older people and their families: key issues in policy and practice/Mike Nolan, Sue Davies, Gordon Grant (editors)
     p.   cm.
  Includes bibliographical references and index.
  ISBN 0-335-20561-5 – ISBN 0-335-20560-7 (pbk.)
  1. Social work with the aged.   2. Aged–Care.   3. Aged–Family relationships.
I. Nolan, Mike, 1953–   II. Davies, Sue, 1958–   III. Grant, Gordon, 1946–
HV1451.W359 2001
362.6–dc21

                                                            00-045271

Typeset by Type Study, Scarborough, North Yorkshire
Printed in Great Britain by Biddles Ltd, Guildford and King's Lynn

For Patrick Nolan 1929–2000
An enduring source of inspiration

Contents

viii *Contents*

Acknowledgements

This book is the product of the first phase of a three and a half year Longitudinal Evaluation of the Educational Preparations of Nurses in the Care of Older People funded by the English National Board for Nursing, Midwifery and Health Visiting. The views expressed are those of the authors and do not necessarily represent those of the Board.

The authors are grateful to the project steering group for their insightful comments and continued support and also owe a debt of gratitude to all those who have contributed and will continue to contribute to the empirical component.

Particular thanks are due to Andrew Booth, Director of Information Services, School of Health and Related Research, University of Sheffield for advice about the literature search strategy, to Kathryn Fish and Helen Mason for secretarial support but especially to Nyree Hulme for endless patience in the production of the final manuscript.

Notes on contributors

Jayne Brown has practised as an RN in neurological rehabilitation, as a district staff nurse and extensively in accident and emergency before moving to the Department of Acute and Critical Care at the University of Sheffield. Her research has included work on stress in nursing and practice nursing roles but now focuses largely on nursing practice in the care of older people.

Sue Davies worked as a health visitor and as a senior nurse within a unit providing services for older people in London before moving into higher education. Her current research interests focus upon the needs of older people in care homes and the development of conceptual and theoretical frameworks to inform practice with older people in a range of care settings.

Claire Ferguson is a research associate currently working on the AGEIN Project. Previous to this she worked in the area of palliative care. Her research interest lies in the area of informal carers and she is currently working on the use of a narrative approach to research with this group of people.

Gordon Grant is Professor of Cognitive Disability at the University of Sheffield. His research interests include family support systems, learning disability and the life course, and empowerment in practice and research.

Elizabeth Hanson is Senior Lecturer in the Department of Community, Ageing, Rehabilitation, Education and Research at the University of Sheffield. She has a strong interest in the palliative care needs of older people and has published in the area of support care.

John Keady is Senior Lecturer in the School of Nursing and Midwifery at the University of Wales, Bangor. John's main interests are in the needs of people with dementia and their carers' and service responses to these needs.

Janet Nolan is a lecturer in nursing at the University of Sheffield. She worked as a health visitor before moving into nurse education. Janet has an interest in health care in the community, in particular the care older people receive from district nurses, practice nurses and health visitors.

Mike Nolan is Professor of Gerontological Nursing at the University of Sheffield. He has a long-standing interest in the needs of older people and their family carers and has published extensively in these areas.

Jane Seymour is a nurse and sociologist. She is a research fellow in the Sheffield Palliative Care Studies Group, which comprises the University Department of Palliative Medicine and the Trent Palliative Care Centre. Jane's particular interests are in older people's understandings of and preferences for, end-of-life care, and the provision of palliative care services to older people with palliative care needs.

Foreword

In 1997, as part of the extensive Research and Development programme evaluating education and practice developments, the Board commissioned a study, the *Longitudinal Evaluation of the Educational Preparation of Nurses in the Care of Older People.* The need to undertake the research arose from a range of sources including previous research completed within the Research and Development strategy, policies which acknowledge the increasing numbers of older people in society and the range and complexity of their needs. The Board is committed to the development of evidence-based professional knowledge to enable nurses working within the multi-professional team to identify and meet the health and social needs of this important client group.

The longitudinal study is due to be completed in summer 2001 and the emergent findings in the final report will be considered in relation to educational policy and practice development.

The Board recognizes the importance of disseminating research findings and is delighted to support the publication of this very informative text, which was presented to the Board in summer 2000. It is commended to all involved in the care of older people and their families including carers, policy makers, managers, educationalists and practitioners in the health professions. Understanding the issues addressed in this book should do much to enhance the quality of practice in the care of older people.

Professor Ron De Witt
Chairman of the Board

Professor Jeff Thompson
Chairman of Research and Development
at the English National Board

Introduction: the changing face of health and social care

Mike Nolan, Sue Davies and Gordon Grant

> Recognising lay knowledge as having an equal part to play in health care decision-making with expert knowledge, provides fundamental challenges to health care professionals.
>
> (Barnes 1999: 25)

The nature of health and social care is changing in fundamental ways. Fuelled by an increasingly well-informed public, expectations of services are rising and 'blind trust' in professional expertise is slowly being eroded, with users and carers actively seeking more equal status (Barnes 1999). While scientific and technological advances increase therapeutic potential, they simultaneously raise tensions, both financial and ethical, about access to treatment and the relative balance between care and cure (Dargie *et al.* 1999). One of the most acute expressions of such tensions arises when the rights and expectations of older people, and particularly vulnerable older people, are considered. Although notions of partnership pervade policy discourse, there is mounting evidence that older people and their carers often remain marginal figures in important decisions about their treatment and care (Audit Commission 1997; Health Advisory Service (HAS) 2000 1998). Indeed recent media attention and consequent public concern about poor standards of care for older people has been such as to cause a significant reorientation of policy, with the new benchmark of quality in the National Health Service (NHS), the National Service Frameworks (NSF) shifting their focus away from 'patients with particular conditions' (Department of Health 1998a) towards more heterogeneous groups such as older people.

The UK government, we are told, will not tolerate substandard care for older people and for the first time the NSF will set national standards which, in moving towards evidence-based care, will recognize that the views and experiences of older people and their carers are an essential part of such evidence (Hutton 1999).

If this is to occur there has to be a dialogue between the abstract knowledge of professionals and the situated knowledge of those on the receiving end of care and services (Barnes 1999). Advancing this dialogue is one of the primary aims of this book. It emerges as the product of the first phase of the AGEIN (Advancing Gerontological Education in Nursing) project, a three and a half year longitudinal study funded by the English National Board for Nursing, Midwifery and Health Visiting. The project itself is evidence of the Board's continuing concern about standards of care for older people and its commitment to advance practice by articulating more clearly the knowledge, skills and attitudes essential to quality care. The ultimate aim is ambitious, to identify an epistemology of practice for those involved in the care of older people.

Such an aim should not be construed as tribal, about protecting or advancing vested professional interests. In tendering for the project we the editors, and all of those contributing to this volume, stated our belief that any epistemology of practice that might emerge should be capable of uniting rather than further distancing disciplines. Most importantly, it should help to reconcile power differentials between professionals and older people and their carers by providing a shared and reciprocal sense of direction and purpose. We therefore adopted a very broad approach to the identification of relevant literature sources (see Appendix).

We considered this essential as recent years have seen the emergence of a number of tensions: within gerontology as a discipline; within policy initiatives designed to address the needs of an ageing society; and among practitioners interested in meeting the needs of older people and their family carers in an holistic but cost-effective manner. Many of these tensions are characterized by a growing interest in the quality of life of older people, particularly the 'oldest old' and how services can maintain a good quality of life in the face of increasing demands and finite resources.

Partnership and empowerment are key themes in the policy rhetoric and coincidentally a number of professions are talking of new 'cultures of care' which are more person-centred. The aim is to educate a generation of 'expert' practitioners who are able to blend tacit and propositional knowledge in creating new ways of working. Yet paradoxically there is growing concern that educational preparation, particularly within health care disciplines, pays scant attention to the needs of older people and that an acute orientation reinforces negative attitudes and predisposes students towards work in more hi-tech areas of care.

To date, gerontology had done relatively little to address such deficits. Bengston *et al.* (1997) suggest that as a discipline gerontology is 'data rich but theory poor' and that there has been little effort to provide a synthesis in key areas. Moreover, they argue that the situation is compounded by the failure to highlight the implications of existing theory for policy and practice. It is precisely these issues that this book seeks to address.

Our primary focus is on factors affecting the quality of life of categories of vulnerable older people and their carers in the context of care delivery in a range of environments. We believe that services will not improve until care, as opposed to cure, is accorded greater value and status and more attention is given to those factors promoting job satisfaction and morale among practitioners.

Care therefore lies at the heart of this book. This reflects a long-standing interest of the contributors in an improved understanding of the nature of care and the interface between those giving and receiving care and between formal and family caring systems. Notwithstanding the diverse and contested nature of care, there is a growing consensus that its complexities cannot be fully appreciated unless due account is taken of the perspectives of all those concerned. Therefore in addition to affording greater recognition to the contribution of those requiring care and support (Nolan *et al.* 1996a), Davies (1998) argues that there is a need to transcend the dichotomies between caregiving (family care), care work (that provided by paid unqualified staff) and professional care. Bringing competence and caring into a new alignment is, she believes, one of the most 'urgent intellectual tasks' for the new century. This book is our own, albeit limited and incomplete, attempt to suggest how such a new alignment might be achieved.

It begins with two chapters intended to 'set the scene'. The first provides a broad overview of issues influencing the quality of life and quality of care for older people and their carers. By integrating these outcome dimensions a framework is introduced comprising six 'senses': a sense of security, continuity, belonging, purpose, fulfilment and significance. It is suggested that these senses provide a potential mechanism for capturing important perceptual and subjective dimensions of 'good care' for both older people and staff. The second chapter explores the notion of 'expertise' and seeks to redefine lay and professional relationships. It highlights different types of knowledge and the emergence of the concept of person-centred care, and the tensions this raises between technical and interpersonal competence.

The subsequent six chapters take a more focused approach and consider the literature on the needs of older people and their carers in six relatively discrete areas. These are acute and rehabilitative care, community care, continuing care, palliative care, mental health in older age and learning disability in older age. The final chapter is a synthesis of the main themes emerging throughout the book. The initial six senses are revisited in the light of the literature and empirical evidence and a more detailed exposition is provided. The senses framework is offered for more rigorous empirical testing and conceptual scrutiny with the hope being that it will offer a mechanism via which to achieve, at least in part, the goal of person-centred care for older people, family and formal carers.

Quality of life, quality of care

Mike Nolan, Sue Davies and Gordon Grant

The findings reported at this congress led us to a profound concern for the future prospects for quality of life of older people everywhere.
(International Association of Gerontology 1998)

The drive to place quality at the heart of the NHS is not about ticking checklists – it is about changing thinking.
(Department of Health 1998a)

Community care policy in the UK reflects contradictory aspirations (simultaneously) promoting resource efficiency and cost effectiveness while advocating a process of needs-led assessment, which provides time for individuals to make their own decisions (Wistow 1995). Nowhere are these tensions more apparent than when the needs of older people, and particularly frail and vulnerable older people, are considered. As there are few precise objectives for community care of older people policy is based primarily on the language of general principles (Henwood 1992). Therefore although higher order concepts such as dignity, independence and autonomy are widely accepted as inherently good, what these actually mean and how they can realistically be achieved is far from clear (Williamson 1992), as such values are 'simple in their expression but highly complex in their translation into behaviour and practice' (Hughes 1995). This complexity is reflected in White Papers on health and social services (Department of Health 1997a, 1998b) and national priorities in both these areas (Department of Health 1998c) which place considerable emphasis on promoting independence and creating a system of 'integrated care' so as to break down the 'Berlin Wall' between various service agencies, and ensure that users and carers become genuine partners. The intention is to focus on what 'really counts' for patients (Department of Health 1997a) so that measures of quality and outcome genuinely reflect the priorities of individuals, their carers and families (Department of Health 1998b). While it is claimed that such policies make sense in both 'human and financial terms' (Department of Health 1998c) more critical analysis suggests that the motivation is economic, fuelled by the desire to relieve pressure on acute and long-term care beds (Hanford *et al.* 1999). Once again therefore current rhetoric reflects the 'language of general principles' and the tensions between humanistic and financial incentives noted by Wistow (1995) are still apparent, indeed exacerbated.

The purpose of this chapter is to explore the above tensions in greater detail and to begin to suggest ways in which general principles might more readily inform policy and practice. The primary focus is on issues to do with the quality of life and quality of care for frail older people. The chapter highlights differences between the perspectives of service providers and older people and outlines a framework which potentially helps to achieve greater convergence.

Outcomes of care for older people

Globally the primary objective of care programmes for older people is to maintain the individual in their chosen environment, most usually their own home (International Association of Gerontology 1998). While some have challenged the taken-for-granted superiority of living in the community (Baldwin *et al.* 1993) there is little doubt that for most people this is their preferred option (Victor 1997). Questions have been raised about the quality of life of frail older people living in the community, and the enrichments or services necessary to promote this (Lawton *et al.* 1995).

Kane (1999) laments the fact that at the beginning of the twenty-first century there is still no clear vision on the responsibilities for, or the potentialities of, home care, beyond keeping someone at home. In order to advance thinking in this area she outlines a range of therapeutic and compensatory interventions and their associated outcomes in a number of domains. Although her analysis is cast primarily in the context of the privately funded system of health and social care operating in the United States her arguments have wider application, particularly in relation to the more subjective and less tangible outcomes. Kane (1999) poses difficult questions about which outcomes are achievable and can be paid for, suggesting that attention is given only to areas such as well-being, autonomy and the promotion of a meaningful life when resources permit. She sees this latter issue as particularly important, believing that there is growing evidence that too many older people, including those living in their own homes, experience a sense of a life not worthwhile; a perception that their value as people has ended.

If the situation is to improve, there is, according to Minkler (1996), a need to adopt a new perspective based on a 'critical gerontology', a value committed approach that seeks not only to understand social ageing but also to change it for the better. Following a similar logic (Kivnick and Murray 1997) contend that services must move beyond remediation and compensation, so that gerontological practice is concerned with identifying, utilizing and enhancing clients' assets. A particular challenge is to transcend traditional welfare structures based on dependency and to address the 'existential doubts' that accompany ageing, in order to help older people maintain or construct a viable identity (Phillipson and Biggs 1998).

Minkler (1996), while acknowledging the importance of structural influences on the ageing process, stresses the need to consider its 'human face' and to reflect upon 'existential meaning in the last stages of life'. In other words, those aspects that help to reinforce a sense of identity and purpose in later life. She questions the largely uncritical acceptance of aims such as promoting independence and successful ageing, arguing that this leads to the stigmatization and disempowerment of those who do not meet the 'criteria' of success. In these 'politically mean-spirited times' she contends that empowerment should be adopted as the unifying concept in critical gerontology, with an attendant focus on interdependence rather than independence and 'power with' as opposed to 'power over' (Minkler 1996).

Others too promote the concept of empowerment (Williamson 1992; Wistow 1995; Clark 1996) and the adoption of a values-based approach to service design, delivery and evaluation (Hughes 1995). While such calls are consistent with the current policy rhetoric they bring into sharp relief the tensions between the desire for quality services to reflect a user perspective and the simultaneous push towards the standardization of outcome measures in health and social care (Sinclair and Dickinson 1998). As Sinclair and Dickinson (1998) note, quality improvement and clinical effectiveness are integrating forces, particularly in the NHS; although there is now more emphasis on the aspirations of older people, the outcome measures most frequently adopted, that is physical functioning and length of hospital stay, remain methodologically and conceptually limited. Therefore while the rhetoric of both politicians and service providers is to 'put the person first', most outcome measures rarely achieve this, raising fundamental questions about 'outcomes for whom' (Bond 1997).

This issue has perplexed providers of health and social care for older people, particularly frail older people, for some time. Challis (1981), for example, identified seven outcome domains for community-based social services for older people: nurturance; compensation for disability; maintenance of independence; morale; social integration; improved family relations; and community development. These domains reflect the need to include both objective and subjective dimensions as highlighted in Kane's (1999) more recent analysis. As Kane (1999) contends, if a critical gaze is applied there is little doubt that, in reality, it is the objective and readily measurable indicators that predominate.

The situation is perhaps even more confused in health care, especially for individuals with chronic illness, where cure is not an appropriate goal (Clark 1996). Tensions about the appropriate goals of care have been apparent since the earliest days of geriatric medicine. There was recognition that the heroic model was not appropriate (Clark 1995) and a functional model in which improvements in physical functioning became the main criteria of success was substituted (Wilkin and Hughes 1986). Therefore despite claims to an holistic approach practice was still dominated by a biomedical construction of ageing (Reed and Watson 1994; Koch and Webb 1996). This had a particularly pernicious impact in long-term care settings where the continued application of a curative or restorative model (Reed and Bond 1991) led to a failure to specify valued goals, so that patients were subjected to 'aimless residual care' (Evers 1991).

The above dilemmas are currently exacerbated by the rising numbers of frail older people living in the community (Victor 1997) and the increased prevalence of chronic illness (Clark 1995). This has led some to call for a paradigm shift in the way that the goals and outcomes of care for older people are conceptualized (Bond 1997), so that the main focus is on quality of life (O'Boyle 1997). Quality of life is viewed as a potentially unifying concept for care services (Renwick *et al.* 1996) and the way in which it is defined and measured is therefore of considerable significance.

Quality of life

With greater recognition that prolonging life at any cost is less important than the quality of life lived (Clark 1995), increasing attention has been given to the way in which quality of life is defined and measured (Brown *et al.* 1996a; Renwick *et al.* 1996; Haas 1999). Indeed quality of life is currently one of the most important outcomes of health and social care, particularly when cure is no longer an option (Martlew 1996; O'Boyle 1997).

While Renwick *et al.* (1996) suggest that quality of life may provide a potentially unifying concept, there is little consensus as to a definition (Bowling 1995b; Farquhar 1995; Hanestad 1996; Haas 1999). Although there is widespread agreement that the concept is multidimensional, and comprises both objective and subjective components (Farquhar 1995; Woodend *et al.* 1997; O'Boyle 1997; Powell-Lawton 1997; Haas 1999) existing measures possess limited validity, particularly when applied to older people. Current approaches exhibit a youthful bias, with the content of most scales being dominated by items of questionable relevance to older people (Stoats *et al.* 1993; O'Boyle 1997; Reed and Clarke 1999a). To compound matters objective criteria figure more prominently than subjective perceptions in most existing measures (Farquhar 1995), usually reflecting taken-for-granted notions of autonomy and independence, operationalized primarily using indices of physical function. Autonomy, it is suggested, has replaced dependence as the main concept underpinning health and social care (Williamson 1992), with some arguing that it currently carries more weight than it can bear (Carson 1995). Autonomy and independence primarily reflect the essential ethic of the American way of life (Trieschmann 1988) with self-reliance being 'lionized' (Kivnick and Murray 1997) by a society that values 'doing' rather than 'being' (Charmaz 1983). Clark (1995) argues that while most authors endorse the importance of quality of life the present overriding emphasis on independence, measured using proxy indicators of Activities of Daily Living (ADL), has to be challenged.

Unfortunately, the importance accorded to ADL is so deeply entrenched that the assumptions upon which such a model is based are rarely recognized, let alone challenged, with Porter (1995) contending that an ADL research tradition dominates the consideration of outcome measurement, especially in health care. Thus a professionally derived conceptualization of quality of life, based primarily on objective criteria, has hegemony (Farquhar 1995; Wistow 1995; O'Boyle 1997; Haas 1999) and if subjective criteria are included they usually reflect the perceptions of researchers (Day and Jankey 1996), with patients' or carers' views rarely being adequately addressed (Chesson *et al.* 1996). The dominance of a professional perspective is a matter of considerable concern as there are often 'striking discrepancies' between the views of professionals and those of disabled people (Loew and Rapin 1994; O'Boyle 1997; Livingston *et al.* 1998; Reed and Clarke 1999a), who frequently hold differing value maps and fundamental perceptions (Clark 1995, 1996). Consequently, as Peters (1995) notes, professionals and users often have a significantly different understanding of the phenomena that initially brought them together.

Discontent with existing approaches to measuring quality of life, which 'lose the human being' (Kivnick and Murray 1997), have led for calls to move beyond 'statistical sophistication' (Bowling 1995a) towards a model which sees the older person as a 'sentient partner' (O'Boyle 1997), and the subject rather than the object of care (Williamson 1992). Incorporating a meaningful subjective element into quality of life measures is a major methodological and conceptual challenge (O'Boyle 1997), as the success of services depend substantially on our understanding of how frailty is perceived and understood by patients and caregivers (Schulz and Williamson 1993).

Numerous authors therefore argue that the fundamental questions in relation to older people are 'what gives life value and meaning?' (Loew and Rapin 1994; Clark 1995, 1996; Hanestad 1996; Prager 1997) and 'what is required to sustain, or if necessary reconstruct, a serviceable sense of self?' (Charmaz 1983; Powell-Lawton, 1997). As noted earlier, existential questions such as 'who am I' are particularly important to a better understanding of later life (Minkler 1996; Phillipson and Biggs 1998). Methodologically this requires a phenomenological approach (Stoats *et al.* 1993; Bowling 1995b; O'Boyle 1997) in order to capture an emic, or insider, view (Peters 1995; Johnson and Barer 1997). Moreover, for older people in particular, quality of life indicators should incorporate a biographical and temporal dimension (Clark 1996) that provides a sense of past, present and future (O'Boyle 1997). This shifts the focus away from an almost exclusively problem orientated model towards a more balanced approach that recognizes both the limitations and potential that ageing presents (Clark 1995; Fontana 1995; Kivnick and Murray 1997; Wenger 1997; Thorne and Paterson 1998). Only in this way will a more sophisticated understanding of what comprises 'successful ageing' emerge (Baltes and Carstensen 1996; Wenger 1997).

Consequently theoretical development is essential to advancing gerontology in general and quality of life in older age in particular, as current approaches to quality of life usually reflect powerful vested interests rather than sound theory (Bond 1997). Indeed quality of life measures are often a-theoretical (Clark 1995; Hughes 1995; Renwick and Brown 1996; O'Boyle 1997); while this is partly due to the lack of consensus on development in old age (Hughes 1995; Bengston *et al.* 1997) others argue that a clearer understanding of what constitutes a good quality of life in older people could be attained if more use were made of existing theories (Hughes 1995; O'Boyle 1997; Wenger 1997).

Theorizing quality of life and successful ageing

Coleman (1997), one of the foremost psychologists of ageing in the UK, believes that to date too little attention has been given to the psychology of ageing and suggests four areas in which further work is needed. These are:

- recognition of the importance of a lifespan perspective
- a consideration of development in later life with a focus on 'ordinary' as opposed to 'exceptional' ageing
- more study of the individual life, moving away from what is statistically 'normal'
- the need to achieve a balance between the third and fourth ages in order to appreciate the existential challenges of frailty.

Coleman suggests that the continued failure to address this latter issue perpetuates a profound failure of meaning. Therefore while early studies on ageing painted a nihilistic picture, currently too much emphasis is placed on people who age exceptionally well (Minkler 1996; Coleman 1997; Thorne and Paterson 1998). For example, Thorne and Paterson (1998), in summarizing trends in research into chronic illness during the 1980s and 1990s, chart the move away from an illness as burden model towards a more positive perception. They caution that the image of the cheerful, existentially transformed person with chronic illness does not necessarily reflect reality for most people.

Nevertheless there is an emerging body of work which suggests that despite the increasing frailty associated with advanced older age, individuals generally manage to sustain a positive view of their quality of life. Such findings are said to represent an 'empirical puzzle' (Brändstädter and Greve 1994), being described as 'counterintuitive' (Johnson and Barer 1997) and therefore in need of further exploration. Authors such as Minkler (1996) argue that there is a need to better understand 'meaning' in later life and that to do so we must transcend the present preoccupation with the state of the body. Only in this way will we learn to appreciate how older people adapt positively to the limitations that ageing inevitably imposes (Loew and Rapin 1994; O'Boyle 1997; Wenger 1997). A number of recent theories offer potential explanations and while each asserts the superiority of its own position there is nevertheless an underlying uniformity suggestive of an emerging consensus. A number of these theories are outlined briefly below.

Coleman (1997) believes that one of the most elegant psychological theories of successful ageing is that proposed by Brändstädter and Greve (1994). Based on considerable empirical work these authors argue that an adequate account of how people maintain a sense of personal continuity and meaning in the face of the multiple losses that often accompany ageing must have three elements:

• It should account for continuity of purpose over time.
• It should be 'biographically meaningful', not focusing solely on the 'here and now' but incorporating past beliefs and values.
• It should discriminate self from others, that is, it must account for individual variation.

Brändstädter and colleagues argue that it is the ability to balance three sets of processes and perceptions which explains how individuals maintain their psychological well-being and sense of meaning and identity in older age. First, there is assimilation, which comprises the efforts people make to maintain their original goals and aspirations. Assimilative activities are most useful when problems are reversible or can be easily compensated for. However, there comes a time when striving to maintain original goals or standards of performance is no longer productive and accommodation is the most effective strategy. Accommodation involves either downgrading or rescaling performance so that it is consistent with available resources, or maintaining levels of performance but in a different area of activity. In order to illustrate these strategies Lundh and Nolan (1996) use the example of a sportsman who plays top flight rugby. As he ages he might strive to maintain this standard by training for increasingly longer periods but running greater risk of injury. While this can be sustained up to a point by what Brändstädter *et al.* (1993) term 'tenacious goal pursuit', this will eventually lead to disappointment. Alternatively, if rugby remains the desired activity then goals could be reappraised so that active involvement is maintained for example, by playing at a lower standard or by a sideways move into refereeing. On the other hand if competing at the top level is the main objective, with the sport itself being less important, then another avenue, for example golf, could be pursued. This has a handicapping system which allows people to compete on more equal terms for considerably longer. Although rather simplistic, this example is nevertheless useful as it illustrates that achieving a balance between accommodation and assimilation occurs throughout life and is not just a function of advanced old age. 'Flexible goal adjustment' is therefore a key process (Brändstädter *et al.* 1993).

The theory also suggests that certain 'identity components' are so central to an individual's vision of themselves, that they cannot easily be relinquished. In these situations a third strategy may be evoked, termed 'Immunization'. This involves individuals selectively interpreting stimuli or events that threaten core identity components, either by playing down their significance or cognitively enhancing their own level of performance. The essence of this theory is that if goals and aspirations are consistent with realistic options then successful ageing is far more likely. Consequently Brändstädter and colleagues argue that accommodation should not be seen as resignation but rather positive adaptation.

While not explicitly following this theoretical approach, other empirical work of a more sociological orientation lends support to this central tenet. Wenger (1997), for instance, suggests that older people who are able to narrow their horizons and accept positively the opportunities available to them report a better quality of life. Similarly, Johnson and Barer (1997) in their extensive longitudinal study exploring how individuals over the age of 85 adjust, found that despite increasing levels of disability, subjective well-being often improved. They argue that social, physical and environmental factors were not sufficient to account for these counterintuitive results and that an adequate explanation had to incorporate an existential element. In other words it must account for how people find positive meaning in their experiences. On the basis of their results Johnson and Barer (1997) suggest that the key is to 'reconstitute a self-concept that is consistent with the realities of later life'. This may mean accepting an element of dependency, actively detaching oneself from certain aspects of life and readjusting definitions and meanings. For instance, while most people in this study considered that they still had a friend, this was often a person who some years ago would probably have been seen as an acquaintance. The similarity between this and Brändstädter's accommodative activities are readily apparent. From such a perspective successful ageing is primarily a process of cognitive readjustment and is best understood on an individual basis, in the context of living a particular life. Therefore Johnson and Barer (1997) contend that relatively 'small interventions' can help to improve perceived quality of life, providing they take account of individual aspirations.

The importance of individual perception is mirrored in Baltes and Carstensen's (1996) explanation of successful ageing. Rather than a normative approach these authors promote an explanation based on understanding personal goals. Underpinned by the belief that a useful framework must account for the variations in losses and gains that older people experience, they propose a 'metamodel' comprising three processes:

Selection	this concept lies at the core of the theory and is about making choices and readjusting 'individual goals'
Compensation	the use of alternative means to achieve a goal
Optimization	enriching and augmenting reserves and resources in order to support selection and compensation.

Baltes and Carstensen (1996) cite extensive empirical evidence from a number of studies, both their own and those of other researchers, in support of the above processes. Notwithstanding variation in terminology and a subtle difference in emphasis, this approach is basically consistent with the work of Brändstädter and colleagues.

Steverink *et al.* (1998) contend that successful ageing is a growing theme in the gerontological literature and a major challenge for social policy. While they acknowledge the contribution of the work cited above, they argue that existing theories do not go far enough and that an adequate explanation of successful ageing has to meet three criteria:

- It must focus on individual behaviour and account for changes in physical, social, cultural and psychological circumstances.
- It needs to identify specific goals linked to general behaviours. In other words there has to be greater clarity as to what is being aimed for.
- Criteria for success need to be specified, in order to know when a goal has been achieved.

They propose what they term a 'Social Production Function Theory' of successful ageing. The central tenet is that individuals are basically resourceful and seek to maximize their well-being within the constraints that they face. To do so involves 'framing' their situation and selecting and substituting goals and activity in the domains of physical and social well-being. Steverink *et al.* (1998) contend that there is a need to maintain both physical and social well being in order to age successfully, with five instrumental goals, two physical and three social, providing routes to success. These are:

- Physical well-being

Comfort	satisfying basic needs and an absence of fear, fatigue and pain
Stimulation	relief of boredom, exposure to novelty, challenge and interesting events.

- Social well-being

Behavioural confirmation	performing, or being seen to have performed, adequately in a certain context

| Affection | being loved by self and others, a perception that others care |
| Status | being valued in comparison to others. |

The relative contribution of the above instrumental goals in achieving overall well-being varies over time and may be culturally determined or influenced by factors such as gender. For instance, status in adult life is often linked to occupation, particularly for men, and may therefore be more difficult to sustain in older age unless an equally valued activity can be substituted. If this is not possible then achieving status may be relegated in importance and social well-being pursued via either behavioural confirmation or affection. The substitution of instrumental goals is possible within but not between domains. In other words, as a minimal requirement for successful ageing at least one of the instrumental goals in the domains of physical and social well-being must be met, Steverink *et al.* (1998) suggest that these are usually comfort and affection. When substitution becomes difficult or impossible individuals will redefine themselves and their aspirations in order to pursue goals that can reasonably be obtained.

Steverink *et al.* (1998) present a number of hypotheses based on their substitution principle for which they provide empirical support from a range of studies. They recognize that important aspects of their theory have yet to be empirically tested, particularly the role of psychological (cognitive) adaptation mechanisms. These aspects do have support from other models such as that of Brändstädter *et al.* (1993), and so some confidence can be placed in the important role of subjective processes in successful ageing.

The above theories emanate from psychology but there is also work of a more sociological nature that confirms and elaborates upon many of the above concepts. For example Ruth and Öberg (1996) stress, as did Coleman (1997), the importance of a biographical approach to successful ageing, arguing that quality of life cannot be understood simply in the light of current circumstances but must recognize the influence of earlier life, so that the 'life lived gives meaning to old age'.

Kivnick and Murray (1997) propose the concept of 'vital involvement' as a key element of successful ageing, highlighting the importance of focusing on both the problems and assets of old people in order to construct an 'ability balance' based on individuals' values, interests, commitments and strengths rather than simply their deficits. Accordingly assessments and information based on this more holistic approach will be more likely to reinforce the values and beliefs that sustain each individual's personal identity.

The importance of maintaining some form of meaningful involvement is also highlighted by Lawton *et al.* (1995), who based on empirical work with frail older people living at home suggest that activity alone is not enough, and that older people also need opportunities to engage in cognitively challenging activities which allow them to demonstrate competence and mastery.

Similarly, writers from a therapy background are increasingly emphasizing the importance of activity being both purposeful and having meaning (Mayers 1995; Trombly 1995). In other words therapeutic activity has a goal or an end point (purpose) but, more importantly, the goal should be valued by the individual concerned. Meaning is therefore essential.

The role of biography, continuity and meaning was highlighted in a study by Nilsson *et al.* (1998). Based on in-depth interviews with over 60 older people, these authors contend that quality of life has little intuitive meaning for older people, since it is a concept imposed on them by researchers and policy makers. On the other hand what makes for a 'good life' in older age is readily understood and older people are able to identify the essential elements. Based on their data Nilsson *et al.* (1998) created a typology of six 'types' of life in older age, ranging from the successful life to the miserable life. Individuals who see themselves as having a 'successful life' do not feel old, even in the presence of disability; they perceive themselves as independent even though they may rely on others; they do not dwell on the past but live life for the present and the future, however short that future may be and they usually have strong personal or religious beliefs. In marked contrast those people who see themselves as having a miserable life speak of being old rather than living; do not feel satisfied with their efforts; have poor relationships with others; and rarely engage in meaningful activity. Nilsson *et al.* (1998) argue that what creates a perception of a 'good life' in older age is not related primarily to objective circumstances but to

- personal relationships – a feeling of embeddedness, usually, but not exclusively, within a family context
- activity – engagement in meaningful activity and a feeling of being needed
- links between past and present lives, where the past is viewed positively, as is the future, no matter how short
- a philosophy of life based on religious or other strong personal beliefs.

Not only is there considerable consistency in all the above accounts, but also similar explanations can be found in related fields, such as chronic illness and learning disability. For instance, Charmaz (1983) suggested that a 'loss of self' was the fundamental form of suffering in chronic illness, and that this was created and sustained by the overriding focus on physical functioning:

> In a society which emphasises doing, not being, those who cannot perform conventional tasks and social obligations lose the very means needed to sustain a meaningful life.
>
> (Charmaz 1983: 191)

More recently Barnard (1995) has argued that autonomy represents one of the most destructive aims for people with chronic illness, and that interventions must instead focus on understanding individual values and aspirations if they are to assist people to relate to life in a way that is responsive to their efforts. He suggests that professionals who thrive on dramatic results and pursue autonomy not only will be disappointed but also do people with chronic illness a disservice.

Within the field of learning difficulties, Renwick and Brown (1996) define quality of life as 'the degree to which an individual enjoys the important possibilities in his/her life'. This reflects their humanistic–existential orientation and their belief that any framework considering quality of life must recognize that while people locate themselves with reference to a place and social group, they also pursue their own goals and make personal choices and decisions.

There are eight basic premises underpinning their model:

- Equal respect for individuals, regardless of their degree of disability.
- Any meaningful view of quality of life must reflect an holistic orientation.
- Quality of life is multidimensional.
- Quality of life is dynamic and interactive, with the relative importance and emphasis given to various components changing over the life course.
- Quality of life arises out of an individual's ongoing interaction with his/her environment.
- Quality of life varies depending on personal value systems, beliefs and interests.
- Quality of life requires a broad conceptualization of health.
- Ultimately the personal perspective of each individual is the most important determining factor.

Having identified these basic premises, Renwick and Brown (1996) suggest that quality of life comprises three major dimensions which they term *being, belonging* and *becoming*. Being is concerned with an individual's physical, psychological and spiritual identity. Belonging addresses the 'fit' between an individual and his/her interpersonal relationships and their physical, social and communal environments. Becoming relates to personal aspirations in terms of purposeful activity, instrumental activity, leisure pursuits and personal growth.

Given the disparate areas in which these varying theories were developed, the degree of congruence between them suggests that there is an emerging consensus about the important parameters of quality of life which recognize that it

- is a multidimensional construct
- comprises objective and subjective elements, each being 'weighted' or given a relative importance dependent upon personal value systems and cultural mores

- is a dynamic and changing entity, varying according to the stage of the life course
- reflects a set of shared concerns but is ultimately a subjective and individual experience.

In the present context the important question becomes 'What are the implications of this consensus for the design, delivery and evaluation of services for frail older people across care environments?' We now move on to consider these.

Promoting quality services for older people

The current emphasis on developing services that reflect the aspirations of users and carers rather than the perceptions of care providers (Department of Health 1997a, 1998b) requires, as the quotation at the beginning of this chapter noted, a change in thinking. Certainly one of the primary goals should be to improve or maintain quality of life and as the above review indicates this means paying more attention to individual values and perceptions. Current conceptualizations of quality life and the measures employed to gauge it appear largely inadequate for the task.

As Kane (1999) argues, we need a more ambitious goal, than simply keeping someone in their own home, if interventions are to promote a meaningful life in older age. Similarly in the UK Redfern (1999) has called for a reconsideration of what constitutes therapeutic activity with frail older people, moving beyond statistical to analytic generalizability.

We believe that there is now sufficient consensus in our understanding of what comprises a 'good life' in older age from a subjective standpoint to provide a degree of analytic generalizability. What is now required is a synthesis of existing theory so as to enhance its practical application.

However, in addition to focusing on what 'counts' for older people and their carers, we believe that quality of care is unlikely to be achieved and sustained unless staff enjoy and value their work. Ageist attitudes and the devaluing of work with older people are still all too apparent in both the health and social services (Health Advisory Service 2000 1998; Social Services Inspectorate 1997). Therefore to be useful a framework must also incorporate staff perceptions and suggest ways in which work with older people can be accorded greater status and value. We offer such a framework below by elaborating on the suggestions of Nolan (1997).

Nolan (1997) was concerned with the lack of a therapeutic rationale for work in long-term care settings with older people and identified six 'senses' which he believed might both provide direction for staff and improve the care older people received. The term 'sense' was selected deliberately to reflect the subjective and perceptual nature of the important determinants of care for both older people and staff. Although in need of further refinement and empirical testing, some of which will be alluded to later (see Chapter 3), we believe that the senses have application beyond long-term care settings, offering a degree of analytic generalizability which can help to inform service development across a range of care environments. A summary of the senses is presented in Table 1.1.

In presenting this framework we would like to make two important caveats. First, its focus on the subjective elements of ageing is in no way intended to deny the importance of structural factors. Rather, as with

Table 1.1 The six senses

A sense of security	
• For older people	Attention to essential physiological and psychological needs, to feel safe and free from threat, harm, pain and discomfort.
• For staff	To feel free from physical threat, rebuke or censure; to have secure conditions of employment; to have the emotional demand of work recognized and to work within a supportive culture.
A sense of continuity	
• For older people	Recognition and value of personal biography; skilful use of knowledge of the past to help contextualize present and future.
• For staff	Positive experience of work with older people from an early stage of career, exposure to role models and good environments of care.
A sense of belonging	
• For older people	Opportunities to form meaningful relationships, to feel part of a community or group as desired.
• For staff	To feel part of a team with a recognized contribution; to belong to a peer group, a community of gerontological practitioners.
A sense of purpose	
• For older people	Opportunities to engage in purposeful activity, the constructive passage of time; to be able to achieve goals and challenging pursuits.
• For staff	To have a sense of therapeutic direction, a clear set of goals to aspire to.
A sense of fulfilment	
• For older people	Opportunities to meet meaningful and valued goals, to feel satisfied with one's efforts.
• For staff	To be able to provide good care, to feel satisfied with one's efforts.
A sense of significance	
• For older people	To feel recognized and valued as a person of worth, that one's actions and existence is of importance, that you 'matter'.
• For staff	To feel that gerontological practice is valued and important, that your work and efforts 'matter'.

Source: Based on Nolan 1997

Minkler (1996), we fully acknowledge their significance but feel there is a need to shed further light on the existential aspects of ageing. Only in this way can we more fully appreciate the importance of subjective components to an understanding of quality of life in older age (O'Boyle 1997) and begin to identify the 'enrichments' that services might reasonably provide (Lawton *et al.* 1995). Second, we do not see the framework as being complete or necessarily inclusive of all potential subjective components. We do believe that it is consistent with the theories previously reviewed and provides a basis for exploring the ways in which services might more fully reflect the experiences and aspirations of older people and their carers. For this to occur, practitioners will need to shed some of their existing professionally derived notions of quality of life and come to 'know' older people and their carers. This raises fundamental questions about what 'counts' as legitimate knowledge and calls for a redefinition of the relationships between older people, their carers and professionals. This forms the subject of Chapter 2.

2

Who's the expert? Redefining lay and professional relationships

Jayne Brown, Mike Nolan and Sue Davies

As highlighted in Chapter 1, empowerment and participation currently figure prominently in the policy rhetoric and practice literatures as one manifestation of the drive towards developing quality indicators which reflect user and carer experiences of health and social care. Moreover the increasing focus on understanding subjective quality of life from a bio-graphical perspective makes it essential that service providers in some way 'know' the person. Couching policy in the language of general principles (Henwood 1992) is problematic, however, and action is needed if such aspirations are to avoid tokenism (McFadyn and Farrington 1997). At a minimum all parties must share a common language and definitions (McFadyn and Farrington 1997), yet this is often not the case in professional and lay interactions; (Clark 1995, 1996). Therefore while 'person-centred care' may be 'writ large' in the policy rhetoric, reflecting the new ethos of service which places the individual and not the provider at the centre (Williams and Grant 1998), realizing such an ethos calls for a reorientation of professional practice (Clark 1995, 1996; Williams and Grant 1998). Clark (1995) argues that professionals must learn to listen to the life stories of older people in a structured, biographical way so as to cultivate an understanding of the experience of illness rather than simply disease (Williams and Grant 1998). Consequently there is much talk of new 'cultures' of care in diverse areas of practice such as dementia care (Kitwood 1997), rehabilitation (Nolan et al. 1997) and long-term care (Henderson and Vesperi 1995), placing considerable emphasis on the relational context (Pincombe et al. 1996; Fagermoen 1997; Mulrooney 1997). Indeed interpersonal relationships are seen to underpin high quality care (Fossbinder 1994; Clark 1996; Janes et al. 1997; Halldorsdottir 1997; Williams and Grant 1998) as a means of accessing and under-standing individual beliefs, values and experiential knowledge. Such relationships raise potential tensions between differing cultures, one professional, the other based primarily on lived experience (Cassell 1991; Clark 1996; Williams and Grant 1998). Reconciling these tensions is essential if person-centred care is to transcend the realm of general principles.

This chapter considers the basis and rationale for interactions between professionals and older people and their family carers. It briefly explores the notion of 'expertise' and calls for a shift in power relations, towards a model of 'power with' or 'power to', rather then 'power over' (Minkler 1996). This requires greater acknowledgement of the 'types' of expert knowledge held by older people and family carers, without denigrating the important, complementary role of professional insights.

Expertise: conflicting paradigms, competing ideologies

Eraut (1994) in a detailed analysis of professional knowledge argues that the essence of professionalism is power based on claims to specialist expertise; the more unique the expertise the greater the power. Until recently the source of such power was the possession of theoretical or propositional knowledge, so called 'know-that' (Ryle 1949). However, the literatures in a range of semi-professions such as teaching, social work and nursing (Benner 1984; Thompson 1995; Schön 1987) and even more established disciplines such as medicine (Cassell 1991) have increasingly questioned the hegemony of theory, arguing that the intuitive, experiential or tacit side of practice, 'know-how' (Ryle 1949), is as least as important.

The result has been an increasingly divisive and, some would argue, one-sided debate (Paley 1996) about the value of experiential knowledge and its relationship to expertise (Dreyfuss and Dreyfuss 1986; Schön, 1987; Benner and Wruebel 1989). Thompson (1995) contends that such disputes are, implicitly at least, primarily about status and the desire of aspiring professions to claim some form of unique knowledge (Nolan *et al.* 1998c). Unfortunately the result is often a polarization of opinion in which theoretical knowledge is increasingly denigrated (Levine 1995) with a growing tendency to 'undermine the rational in favour of the intuitive' (Bradshaw 1995). Those who promote such intuitive knowing often do so using eloquent, if somewhat emotive, metaphors contrasting the 'hard high ground' of technical rationality and the certainty of scientific knowledge with the 'swampy lowlands' and multiple realities of practice (Schön 1987).

Although such arguments are persuasive, Eraut's (1994) penetrating critique exposes a number of limitations, both conceptual and methodological. For example he suggests that Schön's (1987) thesis is based almost exclusively on a consideration of professional creativity and artistry, the type of competence that skilled practitioners sometimes display in 'unique, uncertain or conflicted situations'. Although a valued component of expertise Eraut (1994) contends that context, and particularly time-frame, have been overlooked by many proponents of experiential knowledge. He suggests that there are 'hot' situations which require rapid actions and leave little time for deliberative thought but that conversely there are 'cool' situations where strategic thinking is required. Arguments in favour of intuitive knowledge pay too little attention to these latter situations. Moreover, if the basis of professional skill and competence is primarily intuitive what are the implications of this for multidisciplinary teamwork and communication with clients and carers?

Eraut (1994) believes that arguments about the relative merits of different forms of knowledge are potentially spurious and designed to promote status. Similarly Thompson (1995) calls for professions to move beyond elitism and the pursuit of status and focus their energies on a commitment to developing better services.

Although this brief consideration has simplified a complex situation, current debates have served a number of useful purposes, particularly in promoting greater recognition of lay expertise. First, they have challenged the belief that professional expertise is inherently beneficial (Eraut 1994; Paley 1996). Second, even in disciplines such as medicine, they have highlighted the need to complement science, that part of practice to do with managing the disease, with art or those elements of practice to do with caring for patients as individuals (Cassell 1991). Third, acknowledgement of experiential knowledge has legitimized lay individuals' claims to possess a differing but equally important form of 'expertise'.

In highlighting the knowledge potentially held by frail older people the literature on chronic illness provides important insights, having long argued that 'top-down' models of professional practice (Strauss and Corbin 1988) fail to recognize the differing types of 'work' required in managing long-term illness, thereby ignoring the genuine expertise held by lay people (Strauss *et al.* 1984; Strauss and Corbin 1988). This can have a profoundly detrimental effect on the quality of communication between professionals and disabled people.

For example in a study examining consultations between doctors and patients, Tuckett *et al.* (1985) identified four main foci for their conversations:

- the diagnosis
- treatment and advice
- perceived consequences of the above
- patients' understanding of their treatment.

During detailed observations they found that consultations were one-sided, with little emphasis being given to the latter two areas above. Patients' attempts to clarify their understanding were often ignored and the advice they were given was rarely individually tailored. Tuckett *et al.* (1985) suggested that patients were in many ways already experts about their condition but that doctors generally did not seek their theories. Moreover as doctors believed that the biomedical knowledge they held would be too complex for patients they provided only superficial explanations. On the basis of their work they concluded that there is a need to redefine the role of the doctor in decision making to one of helping patients make their own decisions rather than imposing a decision on them. As Williamson (1992) contends the aim should be to have professional participation in patient decision making, rather than patient participation in professional decision making.

This suggests a considerable reorientation of professional practice and education which currently provides relatively little incentive to take account of the social processes of consultation (Kleinmann 1995). Consequently, the trust that is essential for reciprocal and negotiated relationships can be very difficult to establish or easily compromised (Thorne 1993; Halldorsdottir 1997) and, once lost, may prove impossible to regain (Thorne 1993). There is a need for a more sophisticated understanding of the types of knowledge held by older people and their carers. Fortunately the literature on chronic illness provides some important insights in this regard.

From accounts of individual experiences of chronic illness/disability three themes emerge, which although distinct, share a degree of overlap, suggesting an interactive and dynamic relationship between the *existential, biographical* and *temporal* dimensions of illness/disability.

From an existential perspective, loss of a sense of 'self' has long been recognized as one of the most devastating effects of illness and disability (Blaxter 1976; Bury 1982; Charmaz 1983, 1987; Corbin and Strauss 1988; Robinson 1988; Corbin and Strauss 1991; Beckmann and Ditlev 1992; Carricaburu and Pierret 1995) with Robinson (1988) suggesting that the result is often a 'demolished identity'. Reconstructing a new and equally valued identity is one of the key tasks in adapting to chronic illness (Charmaz 1983, 1987; Robinson 1988), as creating a new sense of 'I' is essential for recovery and adaptation to begin in earnest (Beckmann and Ditlev 1992). This means accommodating to an existential world comprising conflicting feelings of hope, transcendence and despair (Kleinmann 1995).

Living with chronic illness is primarily concerned with 'being' rather than 'doing' (Robinson 1988) but there is scant acknowledgement of the importance of existential factors in the mainstream literature, and consequently the 'judgement, wisdom and ingenuity' that professionals should bring to bear (Strauss *et al.* 1984) is seldom apparent. Barnard (1995) noted that professionals thrive on 'dramatic results' and feel a failure when these prove elusive. He advocated the need to develop the skills of 'empathetic witnessing' in order to help ill or disabled people make sense of their 'existential paradox', caught as they are between an increased awareness of their own finitude and the need to transcend their illness. Others also speak of transcending illness and restoring a sense of living a valuable life

(Gerhardt 1990; Milz 1992; Marris 1996), as only in this way will disabled and chronically ill people achieve a sense of health and wellness (Jensen and Allen 1994; Luborsky 1995) and be able to live life as a 'healthy ill person' (Milz 1992).

Two complementary concepts, also necessary for a more complete understanding of illness or disability, are biography and temporality. Reconstructing a sense of 'I' (Beckmann and Ditlev 1992; Peters 1995) is not possible without reference both to the past and also to a number of potential futures (Gerhardt 1990), and it is often necessary to reconceptualize the past in order to construct a meaningful future (Jensen and Allen 1994; Fife 1995; Kleinmann 1995; Luborsky 1995). One of the most significant effects of chronic illness and disability is that it separates the past from the present and the present from the future, thereby rendering biography 'discontinuous' (Corbin and Strauss 1988). Restoring continuity necessitates a fundamental rethinking of biography and self-concept (Bury 1982), biography in this context serving to unite the existential and temporal dimensions of illness and disability.

There is a clear overlap between many of the ideas in the literature on chronic illness and disability and that on ageing considered in Chapter 1, particularly the importance of understanding subjective meanings from a temporal or biographical perspective. This reinforces the need to 'know the person' if person-centred care is to become a reality. Such a change in emphasis has a potentially profound effect on professional practice, some of the implications of which are considered later.

'Knowing the person'

In considering the rationale for interventions with frail older people, Kivnick and Murray (1997) contend that, although remediation and compensation are important, there is a need for a more holistic focus that enables older people to contribute more actively. They suggest that relationships between older people and professionals should be based on 'interpersonal mutuality'. Similar arguments are advanced by Williams and Grant (1998) who believe that person-centred care requires knowledge of people as individuals, exploring and recognizing their ideas, beliefs and lay knowledge.

Mulrooney (1997) extends the criteria for person-centred care, identifying three attributes:

- respect for personhood
- valuing interdependence
- investing in caregiving as a choice.

These dimensions capture the dynamic and reciprocal nature of person-centred care and largely undermine the notion of 'professional distance'. Clearly while relationships with professionals are different from those with others, for example family and friends, a detached and relatively uninvolved professional stance appears antithetical to a person-centred approach. Mulrooney's last attribute, investing in caregiving as a choice, is perhaps particularly pertinent as there is growing evidence that work with older people remains the least preferred career option and that ageist attitudes still prevail in social and health care (Social Services Inspectorate 1997; Health Advisory Service 2000 1998).

It follows that if person-centred care is to underpin professional practice meaningfully (Rodwell 1996) there is a need for a marked shift in emphasis, so that the client is viewed as an active agent and analyst of their own experience. Such an orientation exposes the limitations of the argument in favour of professional expertise. While Thorne and Paterson (1998) believe that more emancipatory models of care are to be broadly welcomed, these authors caution that the role of an 'outsider expert' should not be entirely denigrated. They argue that there is a need to

> explore the intricate, complex and highly sophisticated skills that comprise professional expertise rather than rushing towards a model in which the professional role is merely to ensure access to services.
>
> (Thorne and Paterson 1998: 176)

They posit that the relative contribution of the 'outsider' expert and 'insider' expert varies over time, depending on the nature of the support required. The need for professionals to work in partnership with disabled people and their carers is consistent with other temporal models of care (Corbin and Strauss 1991; Rolland 1994; Burke 1997) suggesting that professionals must move beyond technical competence to consider the skills and knowledge that they require to deliver person-centred care.

Probably the most detailed consideration of person-centred care is to be found in the nursing literature, with numerous authors promoting such an approach (Fossbinder 1994; Benner and Gordon 1996; Benner *et al.* 1996; Tanner *et al.* 1996; Halldorsdottir 1997; Janes *et al.* 1997; Liaschenko 1997). A number of these authors suggest that knowing the patient as a person allows practitioners to synthesize their understanding of patterns of response to certain illnesses with their knowledge of the individual, in order to identify the 'salient' aspects of a situation (Benner *et al.* 1996; Tanner *et al.* 1996). This synthesis is seen not only to enhance the clinical components of care but also to limit vulnerability and promote dignity. Saliency, that is the ability to identify key aspects of a situation, is seen as one of the core attributes of the gerontological nursing specialist, as indicated in Table 2.1.

Liaschenko (1997) argues that while numerous authors focus on knowing the patient or the person, most of these conceptualizations are still implicitly underpinned by a largely biomedical orientation. In other words knowledge of the person is viewed primarily as a route to a better understanding of their response to illness. Although this is obviously important, particularly in the context of an acute episode, Liaschenko

Table 2.1 Key attributes of gerontological nurse specialist

- *Holistic knowledge and practice* – ability to synthesize a diverse range of knowledge to provide person-centred holistic care aimed at enhancing quality of life.
- *Saliency* – ability to identify key issues of relevance to the older person and select models of care that are interdisciplinary, holistic and person-centred.
- *Knowing the patient* – uses in-depth knowledge of individual and family biographies to work in partnership.
- *Moral agency* – respects and promotes dignity, choice and autonomy to empower older people and their carers.
- *Skilled know-how* – delivery of expert care in an holistic, proficient and fluid way.

Source: Adapted from Ford and McCormack 1999

(1997) believes that other knowledge is required in longer term relationships; knowledge which alerts practitioners to what it is like to live a particular kind of life. She identifies three broad types of knowledge that might inform nursing, and we would suggest health and social care, more widely. These are:

- *Case knowledge*   This comprises biomedical, disembodied knowledge of a particular condition, for instance stroke.
- *Patient knowledge*   This is best viewed as a 'case in context'. In other words information about a person's social circumstances, level of support and so on provide a better understanding of the impact of the 'stroke' and the resources that can be mobilized.
- *Person knowledge*   This is based on understanding 'biographical life' which for Liaschenko (1997) comprises three components: agency, the capacity to initiate meaningful action; temporality, which is related to an individual's pattern of life rather than 'clock time'; space, in terms of how an individual relates to their physical, social and political environments so as to create a sense of 'belonging' somewhere.

Liaschenko (1997) argues that patient and person knowledge are decidedly different and that for 'interventionist' disciplines, that is those which aim to do things to or for people, person knowledge is often essential in order to promote and maintain individual integrity. However, she believes that person knowledge is not appropriate in all contexts.

Eliciting person knowledge takes time and trust and thus case and patient knowledge may be more relevant in situations where the primary aim is to cure a condition and 'move a person out'. Person knowledge is not therefore intrinsically desirable and may be unacceptably intrusive in certain contexts. Conversely person knowledge is usually essential where there is an ongoing relationship, for example in the case of older people with learning disabilities, and its value but also its potentially resource intensive and time consuming nature has to be recognized. For

Liaschenko (1997) this raises political questions, not only for professionals but also for society more generally, about the type of health care that we 'envision'. Person-centred care cannot be manifest unless the skills required are seen as not only legitimate but also important. Liaschenko doubts that this is the case as:

> the kind of attentiveness this [person] knowledge demands is increasingly being seen as fluff, not essential to a vision of health care in which people are cared for only on the basis of case and patient knowledge.

(Liaschenko 1997: 37)

Halldorsdottir (1997) contends that modern day health care has witnessed a separation of competence, that is the delivery of complex technical care, from caring as an affective process, the former being seen as the preserve of the professions and the latter delegated to others. She argues that simply being warm-hearted and having common sense are inadequate, and that good care must combine competence with caring if quality is to be maintained. This requires a model of competence that extends beyond the delivery of excellent technical care, to one which is based upon a more sophisticated understanding of the skills required for a person-centred approach.

Realizing person-centred care

Without devaluing technical competence and care/patient knowledge, it is clear that person knowledge requires differing, but complementary skills and understanding. While these are largely interpersonal skills, the importance of merging such attributes with differing types of knowledge also has to be recognized.

Griffin (1997), for example, argues that if individuals are to be empowered and enabled to use service systems to their best advantage then they need certain forms of understanding. Furthermore if professionals are to facilitate such an understanding they too require a thorough grasp of four types of knowledge:

- *Structural knowledge* of the way the health and social services work.
- *Communicative knowledge* and the ability to interpret the language used by both patients and professionals.
- *Cultural knowledge* and the influence of differing ethnic and racial beliefs on the way that health and illness are construed and the expectations individuals have of service systems.
- *Social knowledge* of the individual, their resources and background.

(after Griffin 1997)

Many of the above are seen as akin to patient knowledge (Liaschenko 1997) but their orientation is different as patient knowledge is intended primarily to alert practitioners to an individual's response to illness, whereas Griffin (1997) suggests that practitioners utilize these four types of knowledge to enable individuals to exert greater control over their situation. This latter approach has a more emancipatory character.

In their analysis Benner and Gordon (1996) distinguish caregiving from caring, arguing that the latter is a form of generalized concern for others. They suggest that caregiving comprises

> Special skills, reflection and activities that allow us to be with and do for another, especially at inconvenient or uncomfortable moments when another human being is needy, weak, vulnerable, recalcitrant and resistant to care, old, ill or dying.
>
> (Benner and Gordon 1996: 41)

Caregiving therefore extends beyond physical expertise and is not simply a technique but a form of responsive interaction. Fossbinder (1994) argues that in order to facilitate such interactions practitioners require interpersonal competence. In her extensive consideration of the literature she identifies a number of domains of interpersonal competence which are summarized in Table 2.2.

While Fossbinder's (1994) arguments are aimed primarily at nurses, they are consistent with Tarlow's (1996) far-ranging analysis of caring in both personal and professional relationships, the attributes of which are illustrated in Table 2.3.

Such frameworks provide important insights into the dimensions of caring relationships, however implicit within them is the ability of the older person to communicate meaningfully. These results say relatively little about how caring can be manifest when there may be communicative or cognitive difficulties, such as following stroke or in older people with learning difficulties or dementia. Caring also requires a context and for older people in contact with health and social services such a context is usually provided by the need for some form of support. As Phillipson and Biggs (1998) contend, traditional models of welfare are usually framed

Table 2.2 Dimensions of interpersonal competence

Translating	informing, explaining, introducing, teaching
Getting to know you	personal sharing, humour, being friendly, 'clicking'
Establishing trust	creating confidence in ability to provide competent care
Being in charge	knowing what to do
Anticipating need	
Being prompt	
Following through	delivering care as promised
Enjoying the job	
Going the extra mile	

Source: After Fossbinder 1994

Table 2.3 Attributes of effective caring

These attributes are seen as prerequisites:
• Having sufficient time
• Being present and prepared to help when needed
• Talking as a vehicle to building and maintaining relationships

These attributes largely determine the quality of caring:
• Sensitivity to the needs of others and the ability to 'notice' when situations change
• Acting in the best interests of another
• Caring as feeling, based on concern or affection
• Caring as doing, to act on behalf of another (when judged appropriate)
• Reciprocity, a negotiated but often tacit understanding of the give and take in relationships

Source: After Tarlow 1996

within a dependency relationship, but as we have sought to demonstrate in this and Chapter 1, the emergence of person-centred care has challenged many assumptions about notions of expertise, who possesses it and the basis for professional interventions. Kleinmann (1995) believes that the key to professional practice is the ability to create a therapeutic narrative with patients and their family. So far we have focused on ways in which such a narrative might be initiated with older people. We now turn attention to interactions with family carers.

Family carers: the unacknowledged experts

Family carers lie 'at the heart of community care' (Warner and Wexler 1998) and it is estimated that they provide approximately 80 per cent of the support needed to maintain frail or disabled individuals at home (Walker 1995a). The recent trends towards empowerment and partnership of older people noted earlier are also apparent in the literature relating to family carers (Askham 1998). Despite the introduction of the Carers (Recognition and Services) Act 1995, which provides carers with a statutory right to an assessment of their needs, several recent studies have suggested that carers often remain marginal figures, rarely consulted or provided with the information and support they require (Fruin 1998; Henwood 1998; Warner and Wexler 1998; Robinson and Williams 1999).

Banks (1999) argues that although carers' issues figure prominently in policy discourse which provides broad statements of general commitment, many inherent contradictions are 'glazed over' and consequently carers' concerns are still not embedded in mainstream thinking. Carers are frequently not offered an assessment and even when they have one practitioners often make implicit assumptions about their capacity and willingness to care and conceptualize carer support in a narrow and restrictive way (Banks 1999). Therefore while it is acknowledged that good assessment is the key to the provision of appropriate and sensitive services (Social Services Inspectorate 1995; Banks 1999) this rarely occurs. Fruin (1998), for example, found great variation in assessment practice and little evidence of explicit and comprehensive assessment frameworks. All too often assessments were based on an implicit mental checklist with many carers being unaware that they were being assessed. Few case files contained an individual profile of carers' needs and review was either infrequent or overlooked altogether.

Widespread concern over the piecemeal and largely inadequate implementation of the Carers Act resulted in the launch of the Carers' National Strategy (Department of Health 1999a), which was intended to mark a 'decisive change' in policy and practice, including proposals that should enable carers to

- choose to care (or not)
- be adequately prepared to care
- receive relevant help at an appropriate stage
- be enabled to care without detriment to their inclusion in society or to their health.

The strategy places particular emphasis on providing support at key transition points, notably at the beginning and end of care and in helping carers develop skills and competencies. Perhaps most fundamental of all is the notion of choice, with the stated intention of the strategy being to 'support people who choose to be carers' (Department of Health 1999a).

Stating such aims is deceptively easy; achieving them is quite another matter. As Twigg and Atkin (1994) suggested, most agencies and practitioners lack a clear rationale for intervening in family care, beyond maintaining carers in their role and thereby implicitly using them as resources. If progress is to be made there is a need for a more holistic approach to meeting carers' needs.

In summarizing the results of a symposium on supporting family carers presented at the World Congress of Gerontology in Adelaide 1997, Askham (1998) called for a broader definition of the purpose of interventions with carers which more fully reflects the growing empowerment approach. According to Askham support can be viewed as any action which helps the carer to

- take up, or decide not to take up, a caregiving role
- continue in the caregiving role
- end the caregiving role.

She also stressed the importance of providing a variety of interventions ranging from training and preparation for caring through information and emotional support, in addition to more traditional instrumental help such as home help or respite care. Responding to such a call requires both a framework for assessment which is sensitive to the dynamic and changing nature of care and a mechanism for collecting the information needed. It is to this area that attention is now turned.

Assessing and responding to carers' needs

As Twigg and Atkin (1994) argue, service agencies and professionals generally lack an explicit rationale for work with family carers and consequently tend to adopt one of four largely implicit models, these are:

- *Carers as resources* – where the aim of support is instrumental, that is to maintain the carer in their role.
- *Carers as co-workers* – where although there is greater recognition of the carers' individual needs the main aim is still instrumental.
- *Carers as co-clients* – where it is difficult to distinguish the needs of the carer from those of the user.
- *The superseded carer* – where the aim of formal services is to replace the carer.

It has been suggested that while these models might be appropriate in given circumstances, none is adequate as a primary basis for intervention (Nolan *et al.* 1996a) as they fail to reflect the ideals of empowerment, partnership and choice which are now being promoted. Underpinning such notions is the principle that all parties bring something of value to an encounter and that views are shared in moving towards a common goal. The literature would suggest that this is often not the case, and that professional and family carers frequently have differing and not necessarily complementary goals and sources of knowledge. For instance, Harvath *et al.* (1994) argue that professionals have what they term 'cosmopolitan' knowledge, that is a generalized understanding of a condition, for example stroke. Carers on the other hand have 'local knowledge' based on their unique understanding of the person having suffered a stroke.

Using Liaschenko's (1997) framework, cosmopolitan knowledge would equate to case knowledge and local knowledge largely to person knowledge. It would seem that the two might most meaningfully come together in helping to shape patient (or client) knowledge. In other words both cosmopolitan and local knowledge are needed in order to understand fully the 'case in context'.

What is required is a model which helps to reconcile potential differences in perception and more adequately reflects the partnership and empowerment approach, recognizing the power differentials that often exist. One such approach is the 'carers as experts' model described by Nolan *et al.* (1996a). Central to this are a number of basic assumptions which can be summarized as follows:

- While an assessment of the difficulties of caring is important, a full understanding will not be achieved unless attention is also given to the nature of past and present relationships, the satisfactions or rewards of caring and the range of coping and other resources, such as income, housing and social support, that carers can draw upon.

- The stresses or difficulties of care can best be understood from a subjective rather than an objective perspective. This means that the circumstances of care are less important than a carer's perception of them.
- It is essential to consider both a carer's willingness and ability to care. Some family members may not really want to care but may feel obliged to do so. Conversely while many family members may be willing to care they may lack the necessary skills and abilities.
- While recognizing the importance of services such as respite care, in-home support and so on the primary purpose of the 'carers as experts' approach is to help carers to attain the necessary competencies, skills and resources to provide care of good quality without detriment to their own health. In this context helping a carer to give up care is a legitimate aim.
- 'Carers as experts' recognizes the changing demands of care and the way in which skills and expertise develop over time. A temporal dimension is therefore crucial, and this suggests varying degrees of 'partnership'. For carers new to their role professional carers are likely to be 'senior partners' in possession of important knowledge of a 'cosmopolitan nature' which is needed to help the carer understand the demands they are likely to face. Conversely experienced carers, many of whom will have learned their skills by trial and error, often have a far better grasp of their situation than professionals and acknowledgement of this is vital to a partnership approach. At a later stage the balance may shift again so, for example, if it is necessary to choose a nursing home, carers may go back to a 'novice' stage, probably never having had to select a home before. They will therefore need additional help and support. Recognizing and achieving such a balance is the crux of the 'carers as experts' model.

Others have also noted the importance of a temporal dimension in responding to carers' needs and the change in emphasis over time which determines whether the professional or carer is seen to hold 'expert knowledge' (Hasselkus 1994). Complementing this picture is the growing awareness of issues to do with caregiving competence and how family carers can be assisted to care 'well' (Schumacher *et al.* 1998). All too often, however, caregiving is a 'solitary journey' with little recognition that carers are usually novices in providing complex physical care and are frequently ill prepared for the longer term consequences of caring (Boland and Sims 1996). How such a 'solitary journey' might become a more shared pursuit is elaborated upon in the remaining chapters.

In this chapter we have explored the recent move towards empowerment and partnership with older people and carers and the implications of such developments for what 'counts' as valid knowledge and who can legitimately claim 'expertise'. In so doing many of the themes from the initial chapter have been reinforced, particularly the importance of sub-jective perceptions and meanings to a better understanding of the com-plex needs of older people and their carers. It is apparent that as needs change over time, so too must the type of professional support that is provided. Responsive and flexible services must take full account of this temporal dimension if quality care is to be provided. The following six chapters will consider the needs of older people and their carers in differ-ing contexts, and many of the issues we have identified in Chapters 1 and 2 will appear again in varying guises. In Chapter 9 these disparate elements will be brought together to try to advance policy, practice and education for all those who work with, or are concerned about, older people and their carers.

3

Acute and rehabilitative care for older people

Mike Nolan

Patients, families and carers should:

> Expect the best of care in acute hospitals. Older people have a right to services provided by staff with expert knowledge and skills, and the facilities that will best meet their needs.
>
> (Health Advisory Service 2000 1998: 68)

The government should

> Maintain the focus . . . on issues surrounding the care of older people in acute hospitals, and elsewhere. They have been a neglected group for too long and the government is right to want to make them a priority.
>
> (Health Advisory Service 2000 1998: 71)

> It is a hard fact that aside from any humanitarian arguments, one of the main forces driving the development of rehabilitation services for older people remains the need to relieve pressure on acute and long term care beds.
>
> (Hanford *et al.* 1999: 16)

The vulnerability of older people in acute hospital environments has been recognized for some time (Gunter 1983) and reaffirmed recently (Health Advisory Service 2000 1998) with some commentators arguing that a culture of 'inhumane care' exists (Koch and Webb 1996) or at the very least that practice is dominated by ritual and routine (McCormack and Wright 1999). A number of reports have highlighted a range of concerns about the health care of older people generally and acute hospital care in particular (Audit Commission 1997; Health Advisory Service 1997; Health Advisory Service 2000 1998), and while the situation is not yet considered, 'parlous' distinct and identifiable problems nevertheless exist including

Table 3.1 HAS 2000: identified deficiencies in care of older people

---

- Delays in admission
- Poor physical environment, lack of basic equipment and supplies
- Staff shortages and over-reliance on junior staff, too few specialist therapists
- Non-availability or poor quality of food and drink
- Lack of attention to feeding and nutrition, insufficient assistance and poor communication during these aspects of care
- Limited privacy and dignity, especially on mixed sex wards
- Pressured staff demonstrating poor attitudes and communication skills
- Failure to negotiate the boundaries of care, mutual expectations unclear
- Occasional difficulties in staff–patient interactions
- Continued difficulties around discharge exacerbated by poor communication between professionals, lack of information to patients and insufficient or inadequate community services

---

Source: Adapted from HAS 2000 1998

inconsistencies in practice, inequalities in care and lack of proper assessment (Health Advisory Service 1997). Many of these difficulties have been attributed to the emphasis on rapid patient throughput (Audit Commission 1997; Health Advisory Service 1997), with the length of hospital stay of older people having fallen by 45 per cent between 1992 and 1997 (Audit Commission 1997). Additionally there have been recent concerns of a more fundamental nature about the lack of basic dignified care for older people in acute hospitals, exacerbated by restrictive care practices and ageist attitudes (Health Advisory Service 2000 1998). The report of an independent inquiry into the acute hospital care of older people convened by the then Secretary of State for Health, Frank Dobson, concluded that while good practice exists there are serious deficiencies in the standard of care for older people. These are summarized in Table 3.1.

How this situation might be improved forms the substance of the initial part of this chapter. Subsequently the focus shifts to consider the present policy of promoting independence among older people (Department of Health 1998b, 1998c; Health Advisory Service 2000 1998) and the consequent renewed interest in rehabilitation (Nocon and Baldwin 1998; Sinclair and Dickinson 1988; Hanford *et al.* 1999). Building on the arguments presented in Chapters 1 and 2, the tensions between professionally derived visions of rehabilitation and those of older people will be explored and the implications for the design and delivery of services considered.

Acute hospital care: back to basics

In their report chronicling the often poor care that older people receive in acute hospital environments, the Health Advisory Service 2000 (1998) team identified three sets of factors thought to exert considerable influence. These were:

- knowledge, skills and attitudes of staff
- general cultural issues
- resources and how they are used.

It is clear from Table 3.1 that there are often inadequate resources, both human and material, to provide care to the standard required. The reliance on junior staff was a particular concern, also noted in other analyses of the health care older people receive (Health Advisory Service 1997). This situation is exacerbated by the difficulty in recruiting sufficient staff to work with older people, this area of care often being the least preferred career option (Hogstel and Cox 1995; Stevens 1997; Davis 1997; Fulmer and Abraham 1998; Health Advisory Service 2000 1998; Stevens 1999). This is a cause for considerable concern as staff are unlikely to be attracted to, or remain in, an area of work which has little perceived status, and is not valued sufficiently (Lawrence *et al.* 1996). However, attention to resource issues, although important, is unlikely to improve the quality of care unless a positive culture exists and staff have the necessary knowledge and skills. There is much contemporary evidence to suggest that both the culture of care in acute hospital environments and the knowledge and skills of staff are not conducive to providing high quality care to older people (Health Advisory Service 1997; Health Advisory Service 2000 1998).

There is growing recognition that ageism can be found at all levels of the health service (Health Advisory Service 2000 1998), with the report by Age Concern (2000) providing clear indications of how pervasive ageist attitudes are. To compound matters too high a priority is still placed on rapid throughput and discharge from hospital (Health Advisory Service 1997; Health Advisory Service 2000 1998) with a consequent tendency to pander to the numbers game rather than promote high quality care (Health Advisory Service 2000 1998). The government itself is now alert to this and, in principle at least, acknowledges the need for change: 'For too long the emphasis has mainly been on counting numbers; of measuring activity; of logging what could be logged; but this ignored the needs of patients' (Department of Health 1998a: 2).

The emphasis on 'counting numbers' has a particularly deleterious effect at the time of hospital discharge when inadequate coordination and liaison between service agencies means that older people and their carers often do not get the help and support they need (Audit Commission 1997; Health Advisory Service 1997; Department of Health 1998b; Health Advisory Service 2000 1998).

Perhaps an even more telling indication of the need for a change in culture is the failure to prioritize and deliver 'basic dignified nursing care' in important areas such as assistance with washing, dressing, feeding and toileting (Health Advisory Service 2000 1998). As highlighted in Chapter 2, interpersonal relationships are essential to person-centred care and it is the delivery of so-called 'basic' care that provides the context for most interactions in acute care environments (Gibb and O'Brien 1990; Grainger 1993; Baer and Gordon 1996; Hudson and Sexton 1996; Hektor and Touhy 1997; Janes *et al.* 1997). The lack of value and status associated with basic, as opposed to technical, care has a negative effect on a number of fronts. Not only do important physical needs remain unmet but the inherent opportunities to foster interpersonal relationships during care delivery are often not realized (Gibb and O'Brien 1990; Granger 1993; Baer and Gordon 1996). Therefore if standards are to improve it is important that both technical and interpersonal competencies are cultivated. The dynamic and reciprocal relationship between these two facets of care was highlighted by Davies *et al.* (1999) in their study examining factors which promote the dignity of older people in acute hospital environments.

This study comprised both an extensive consideration of the literature and detailed case studies in hospitals which had been nominated by older people, or their advocacy groups, as providing high quality care. Both the literature review and empirical component of this study will inform this chapter. In synthesizing the literature relating to dignity and older people in acute hospital environments Davies *et al.* (1999) identified a number of important components, summarized in Table 3.2.

For the present purpose the third point in Table 3.2 is particularly instructive, suggesting that qualified practitioners should be involved in delivering both technical and 'basic' care to the highest standard. Unfortunately it seems that there are often considerable deficiencies in both these areas.

Table 3.2 Key themes from the literature review

- Dignity, although difficult to define, is essentially about feelings of personal worth and identity and is necessary for a good quality of life. Both dignity and quality of life are basically subjective phenomena requiring that practitioners understand the values and preferences of older people. In other words there is a need to 'know' the patient.
- 'Knowing' the patient is based on a personal, professional relationship appropriate to a given context of care. The quality of this relationship appears fundamental to the delivery of optimum care.
- In an acute environment, direct care delivery provides the main purpose for staff–patient interaction. Competent technical care is essential but the value of fundamental personal care must be more fully acknowledged.
- Involvement in direct personal care provides experienced practitioners with opportunities to promote dignity while making skilled assessments of patient need. Standards of care required of others are also made explicit by such actions.
- 'Zero tolerance' of poor care is best achieved via clearly communicated expectations in a supportive rather than punitive culture.
- Promoting and maintaining best practice requires both personal commitment and organizational support, with a certain minimum level of resources.

Source: Davies *et al.* 1999

Delivering competent technical care

In an acute care environment, where cure or restoration is the primary aim the importance of good technical care is obvious (Davies *et al.* 1999). Older people, who often have multiple pathology, however, challenge the acute medical model, requiring attention to a diverse range of both psychological and social factors. Comprehensive assessment of individual need is therefore seen to underpin high quality care (Health Advisory Service 1997; Francis *et al.* 1998; Health Advisory Service 2000 1998; Kresevic *et al.* 1998; McCormack and Ford 1999a). Unfortunately, a number of recent reports suggest that, while the importance of assessment is recognized, holistic approaches are rarely achieved (Health Advisory Service 1997; Health Advisory Service 2000 1998; McCormack and Ford 1999a).

All too often the pivotal initial assessment is left to junior medical or nursing staff, who either focus on medical aspects or concentrate on completing the documentation (Health Advisory Service 1997). The situation is exacerbated by a lack of conceptual clarity as to the purpose of assessment, for although there may be a plethora of quality guidelines and standards these are often ignored as they fail to incorporate the perspective of individual service providers (Health Advisory Service 1997). Moreover staff may lack the knowledge and skills required to conduct detailed assessments in important areas such as continence and swallowing (Health Advisory Service 2000 1998). Such deficits in assessing the technical components of care are often compounded by inadequate social assessments where ageist attitudes can result in limited expectations of the willingness and ability of older people to participate fully and an uncritical acceptance of social isolation and depression as natural consequences of ageing (Social Services Inspectorate 1997).

A consideration of the nursing literature in acute hospital care identifies a range of areas of care in which it is suggested that nurses should be able to undertake a comprehensive assessment and also highlights that such skills are often inadequately developed. A summary of some of these areas is presented in Table 3.3.

Although not intended to be exhaustive, Table 3.3 is indicative of the diverse areas of technical care in which it is argued that nurses should be able to conduct skilled assessments. These skills are frequently deficient, however; assessment of continence provides a case in point.

The HAS 2000 (1998) report concluded that the assessment of continence should be a core nursing skill, a point reaffirmed in Table 3.3. In a synthesis of the available literature Smith (1997) concluded that promotion of continence is most often seen as the responsibility of nurses and highlighted, as do others (Dowd and Campbell 1995; Hancock *et al.* 1996; Resnick *et al.* 1996) the central role of assessment. Schultz *et al.* (1997) consider that nurses in acute care settings are ideally placed to identify continence problems, arguing that 40 per cent of acute care patients of all ages (most usually women) have a degree of incontinence.

Table 3.3 Indicative areas in which nurses should be able to conduct skilled assessments

• Restraint use	Malassiotis and Newell 1996; Bryant and Fernald 1997; Cruz *et al.* 1997
• Risk of falls	Gluck *et al.* 1996; Reece and Simpson 1996; Turkoski *et al.* 1997
• Promotion of continence	Dowd and Campbell 1995; Connor and Kooker 1996; Hancock *et al.* 1996; Resnick *et al.* 1996; Smith, 1997; Schultz *et al.* 1997; HAS 1999
• Constipation	Moore *et al.* 1996; Francis *et al.* 1998
• Nutrition	Tierney 1996; Perry 1997; HAS 2000 1998; Francis *et al.* 1998
• Pain	Forrest 1995; Closs 1996; Simon 1996
• Care of skin	Hamilton and Lyon 1995; Wilkes *et al.* 1996
• Care of feet	Turner and Quine 1996

They estimate that only 10 per cent of this 40 per cent are identified in the nursing notes, however, as patients very rarely report symptoms unless they are asked directly. The limited attention that nurses give to promotion of continence in acute care is reported in a number of studies (Dowd and Campbell 1995; Connor and Kooker 1996; Hancock *et al.* 1996), possibly as nurses tend to see this aspect of care as stressful, frustrating and time-consuming (Connor and Kooker 1996). Moreover, due to deficient knowledge in key areas (Hancock *et al.* 1996; Smith 1997), nursing interventions often lack coherence and consistency (Dowd and Campbell 1995), with either catheters (Dowd and Campbell 1995) or incontinence pads (Connor and Kooker 1996) frequently being used inappropriately as the treatment of first choice.

Although continence difficulties are not confined to older age, it is apparent that more attention to those aspects of care detailed in Table 3.3 has the potential to improve considerably the quality of care older people receive in hospital.

McCormack and Ford (1999a) have suggested that assessing the needs of older people is a 'global challenge' and while they acknowledge the importance of a structured approach they caution against the wholesale adoption of standardized measures that lose the 'uniqueness' of the individual and erode the role of professional decision making. They argue that a person-centred assessment should incorporate three elements comprising the individual's biography, standardized measures and professional judgement. This once again highlights the tensions between the objective and subjective dimensions of care and the need to undertake an individual assessment. Such tensions are increasingly evident in the policy literature, with calls to move away from a 'one size fits all' model (Department of Health 1998b) while simultaneously promoting the standardization of outcome measures (Sinclair and Dickinson 1998).

Within the context of acute care, the work of McCormack and Ford (1999a) reaffirms the importance of biography and interpersonal relationships, the latter area in particular being identified as central to the delivery of high quality care which maintains the dignity of the older person in acute hospital environments (Davies *et al.* 1999).

Promoting dignity in acute hospital care

The impetus behind the independent inquiry into the acute hospital care of older people conducted by Health Advisory Service 2000 was a series of newspaper articles in 1997 which highlighted concerns about the lack of basic dignified nursing care received by older people, with the Health Advisory Service 2000 (1998) report reaffirming this conclusion. In an effort to identify factors that contribute to maintaining the dignity of older patients in acute environments, Help the Aged and the Order of St John's Trust commissioned a study of hospitals which older people had nominated as providing high quality care (Davies *et al.* 1999).

Following a review of the literature and detailed case studies, Davies *et al.* (1999) identified four key principles that appear to underpin good practice:

- Valuing fundamental practice – ensuring that the care needs of older people, particularly in areas such as personal hygiene, nutrition and continence are accorded a high priority and that senior staff are involved in direct care delivery.
- Fostering stability while embracing challenge – working to create a stable ward team and an environment in which staff feel free to innovate and question practice.
- Establishing clear and equitable therapeutic goals – ensuring that older people have the same access to care and interventions as do younger people and that agreed goals of care are negotiated with older people and their carers.
- Commitment to an explicit and shared set of values – having a philosophy of care shared by all staff, which clearly identifies the standards of care expected.

In summarizing those factors which shape the experience of care for older people, their family carers and staff, Davies *et al.* (1999) adapted the six senses outlined in Chapter 1, and in applying these to an acute care context they identified how such senses can be created and sustained. Their suggestions are summarized in Table 3.4. The dynamic and reciprocal relationship between those factors necessary to promote the senses and achieve a positive culture of care for older people in acute hospital environments is captured in Figure 3.1.

The conclusions reached by Davies *et al.* (1999) are consistent with the results of another study which examined the attributes of quality hospital care identified by both patients and nurses (Redfern and Norman 1999).

Table 3.4 Factors shaping the experience of 'care' for older people, their families and staff

Factors creating a sense of	For older people and their families	For staff
Security	Rapid access to a hospital bed when needed Provision of regular, clear information Visibility of nursing staff, senior staff delivering care and central nurses station ensuring that staff are visible Access to 'experts' such as medical consultants and clinical nurse specialists Regularly asking the older person how they feel Risk assessment in negotiation with the older person Support after discharge, e.g. telephone calls, discharge support	Structured mechanisms for clinical supervision and mentorship Experienced staff available for role modelling and problem solving Freedom to challenge poor practice without censure Known boundaries within which to operate Having clear and explicit goals
Significance	Equity of access to medical/therapy care Being involved in care planning and evaluation, e.g. bedside handover, biographical assessment Resources invested in making the environment comfortable and attractive	Investment in personal professional development Opinions valued and listened to Adequate equipment to carry out role Work with older people valued and recognized as important
Belonging	Staff using patient's preferred name Recognition of importance of relationships with other patients Families encouraged to participate in care as appropriate Being treated like family Having designated members of staff to coordinate care Flexible visiting times Tea and coffee available for patients and visitors	Core team of stable staff Blurring of roles Clear sense of belonging to a team Strategies for keeping staff informed, e.g. team briefing, computerized information systems
Purpose	Regular meetings with staff to discuss progress Self-medication programmes Use of care contracts Mutually agreed goals of care. Being a genuine partner in planning and evaluation	Clear therapeutic rationale for care Investing resources in creating effective leadership Regular appraisal and goal setting for all staff All staff encouraged to review practice and suggest improvements, e.g. critical incident audit

Table 3.4 Continued

Factors creating a sense of	For older people and their families	For staff
Continuity	Team nursing/named nursing as the system for organizing care Wards having designated therapy staff Access to schemes aimed at enabling an older person to avoid hospital admission unless absolutely necessary, e.g. Rapid Response scheme Continuity of support following discharge Partnership programmes involving family carers in caregiving Communication sheets to assist discharge Phone calls after discharge Liaison with home care services Staff taking time to get to know the older person	Team nursing/named nursing as the system for organizing care Wards having designated therapy staff Integrated multidisciplinary documentation encouraging continuity of communication Limiting the number of medical teams providing care to one ward Explicit process for inducting new members of staff
Achievement	Being involved in review of progress Feedback Evaluation carried out with the older person Care plans and progress sheets accessible	Recognition of effort, e.g. award schemes Designating additional responsibilities, e.g. link nurse roles Being able to provide best possible care

Source: Davies *et al.* 1999

Although Redfern and Norman (1999) highlighted some differences between the perceptions of patients and nurses, there was also a great deal of consistency with a therapeutic ward atmosphere, therapeutic relationships and attention to emotional needs being signalled out as the three most important indicators of quality by both groups, albeit in a slightly differing order. Conversely being disrespectful, a non-therapeutic environment and insensitivity to vulnerability were seen as important indicators of poor care. Among the key themes to emerge from this study were the need to establish a therapeutic context and the importance of staff displaying sensitive attitudes.

Therapeutic context was determined largely by good facilities and adequate staff; a friendly and welcoming atmosphere, with staff having time to address patients' concerns; an element of continuity, but the absence of a rigid routine; good multidisciplinary working, especially at discharge. Sensitive attitudes were demonstrated by staff who showed patients respect and maintained their dignity; established therapeutic relationships based

Prerequisites

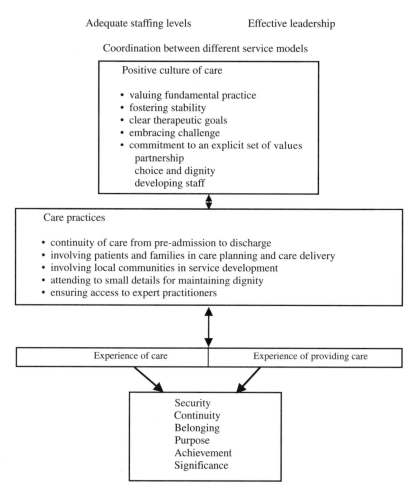

Figure 3.1 Factors promoting and sustaining excellence in the care of older people
Source: Davies *et al.* 1999

on concern, affection and humour as indications of genuine interest in patients; saw patients as individuals rather than work objects; created a sense of emotional security; gave patients as much control as possible; and helped to boost morale by the constructive passage of time.

The similarity between these conclusions, those factors identified in Table 3.4 and the senses outlined in Chapter 1 are readily apparent, highlighting their potential for analytic generalizability (Redfern 1999).

Furthermore as Redfern and Norman (1999) contend, their work is supported by other emerging theories, in particular those of Irurito (1996) and Fossbinder (1994). Irurito (1996) for example argues that quality care requires a combination of technical proficiency (firm hand care) and interpersonal skills (soft hand care), with Fossbinder (1994) elaborating further on the dimensions of interpersonal competence as summarized in Chapter 2 (see Table 2.2).

Clearly therefore the literature on acute hospital care reaffirms the central role of interpersonal and subjective elements in enhancing our understanding of what constitutes quality care for older people, a point which is further developed when the literature on rehabilitation is considered.

Rehabilitative care

Rehabilitation has been described as the 'missing' element in the health and social care of older people (Audit Commission 1997); a number of reports have confirmed that rehabilitative services are particularly underdeveloped in relation to older people (Robinson and Batstone 1996; Baker *et al.* 1997; Sinclair and Dickinson 1998). Although rehabilitation has not traditionally figured prominently in policy discourse, this has changed with rehabilitation having become very topical (Nocon and Baldwin 1998; Sinclair and Dickinson 1998; Hanford *et al.* 1999). It remains to be seen if this recent change in emphasis will benefit older people. The purpose of this section is to explore current conceptualizations of rehabilitation and to consider if they are consistent with the needs of older, and particularly frail older, people.

The promotion of independence is presently one of the main aims of both health and social care policy (Health Advisory Service 2000 1998; Department of Health 1998b, 1998c) an emphasis which has rekindled interest in the concept of rehabilitation. In their analysis of recent policy developments, Hanford *et al.* (1999) suggest that several government documents, as well as non-governmental reports, such as the Royal Commission on Long-Term Care (1999), highlight the importance of rehabilitation, especially for older people. In addition to the promotion of independence the development of a more integrated approach to care is one of the main drivers underpinning current policy (Hanford *et al.* 1999). As a consequence rehabilitation is now seen as 'everybody's business' with a much greater role for social care practitioners. In moving towards integrated care a number of structural and other changes are now being introduced, for example, the development of joint investment plans, health improvement programmes and primary care groups (Hanford *et al.* 1999). Although expressing some concern that the inherent risk of seeing rehabilitation as 'everybody's business' is that it might end up as 'nobody's business', Hanford *et al.* (1999) consider that rehabilitation for older people should improve as a result of current developments, due to a clearer focus and the delivery of more integrated services. The extent to which older people actually benefit depends in no small measure on the way in which the aims and purposes of rehabilitation are conceptualized, with Robinson and Batstone (1996) arguing that informed debate about rehabilitation has been hampered by the lack of an agreed definition, suggesting that greater clarity will not be achieved until rehabilitation is clearly distinguished from other services.

A number of authors have highlighted the difficulties of achieving a uniform definition of rehabilitation (Walley 1986; Waters 1987; Beardshaw 1988; Waters 1991; Tallis 1992; Keir 1996; Waters 1996) and many commentators either fail to provide a definition or else assume a consensus (Waters 1996; Waters and Luker 1996). To compound such difficulties many definitions are accepted implicitly, uncritically or both.

In order to achieve greater consistency, Nocon and Baldwin (1998) undertook a review of the available literature on trends in rehabilitation policy. They concluded that the main aim of rehabilitation is restoration, either of function or role and that it is an emphasis on restoration that distinguishes rehabilitation from primary prevention and maintenance. In order to be effective rehabilitation must be responsive to users' needs and wishes; involve multidisciplinary and multi-agency working; be available when required; and have a clear purpose and goals that distinguish it from other processes (Nocon and Baldwin 1998). However, the primary distinguishing characteristic of rehabilitation is its focus on restoration.

Building on this review Hanford *et al.* (1999) state that the King's Fund defines rehabilitation as an often complex process which enables individuals after impairment by illness or injury, to regain, as far as possible, control over their lives. Rehabilitation is seen to have the following characteristics:

- It is time-limited.
- It is usually a function of services, not necessarily a service in its own right.
- It involves a range of clinical, therapeutic and social interventions.
- It is aimed at restoring an individual's physical and mental capabilities to the optimum level possible.
- It helps individuals to recover social roles that are important to them.
- It is often delivered in a range of settings, including the hospital and the community.
- It should involve the patient and family carers in decision making.

It should be noted that most of the policy and practice literature consulted was professionally derived and this largely accounts for the importance placed on seeing rehabilitation as a restorative time-limited intervention. Such a definition is not necessarily consistent with the views of patients and their carers. Nolan *et al.* (1997) in their extensive comparison of the professional literature on rehabilitation and the views of disabled people themselves, suggest the existence of two paradigms of rehabilitation, which they term the Restricted Isolated Model and the Comprehensive

Integrative Model, each comprising a series of continua, as illustrated in Figure 3.2.

While Nolan *et al.* (1997) argue that neither model probably exists in its pure form, services most closely approximate to the Restricted Isolated Model, with its finite, time-limited emphasis in which success is defined largely by a quantifiable, measurement-orientated approach. In contrast the Comprehensive Integrative Model, derived mainly from the literature relating to the perceptions of disabled people, incorporates a temporal dimension with a focus on the biographical and existential implications of disability. The tensions between these models are tellingly illustrated when the outcomes of rehabilitation are considered.

Restricted Isolated Model		Comprehensive Integrative Model
• Physical orientation	←——→	• Incorporates biographical/existential elements
• Focus on impairment/functional aspects of disability	←——→	• Addresses handicap at individual, community, environmental and societal levels
• Finite, time-limited, emphasis on acute care,chronicity neglected	←——→	• Temporal/longitudinal emphasis, chronicity important
• Outcome/effectiveness driven, economic concerns predominate quantifiable, measurement orientation, static and a-contextual	←——→	• Expanded range of outcomes, incorporation of subjective indicators, includes process variables, dynamic and contextual
• Hospital orientated	←——→	• Includes all environments
• Mainly reactive, secondary prevention	←——→	• Proactive, primary prevention seen as important
• Individualistic focus on patients' functional ability	←——→	• Perspective of family unit seen as important
• Fragmented, ad hoc, service provision and follow-up	←——→	• Coordinated, seamless provision
• Professional (medical) hegemony on expertise and power, interventions of little relevance to daily reality/personal meanings of disabled people/carers, disempowering	←——→	• Expertise/power vested with disabled people/ carers, interventions high/relevant to daily reality/ personal meanings, empowering
• Dominant, western cultural ethos, male orientated, problem solving, personal autonomy	←——→	• Recognizes issues of gender, culture, ethnicity, interdependence, community values
• Methodologically blinkered, theoretically restricted	←——→	• Methodologically and theoretically eclectic
• Experimentally and empirically driven	←——→	• Pluralistic models valued

Figure 3.2 Rehabilitation: contrasting models
Source: Nolan *et al.* 1997

Outcomes of rehabilitation

Complementing the review of developments in rehabilitation policy (Nocon and Baldwin 1998), Sinclair and Dickinson (1998) conducted a systematic review of the evidence base to support rehabilitation practice. Mirroring the conclusion of Nocon and Baldwin (1998) their study highlighted a number of consistent themes, including a greater emphasis on the views of users and carers and a shift towards rehabilitation in a community context. A particular focus of this second review was on outcome measures, with the authors arguing that there is a need for a standardized approach in order to facilitate 'easy pooling' of the results of differing trials and to 'encourage further systematic reviews with even greater impact and meaning'.

Given the importance allocated to 'meaning', it is perhaps paradoxical that the outcome measures most frequently adopted appear to have relatively little 'meaning' for older people and their carers. As a result of their review, Sinclair and Dickinson (1998) concluded that there is a need for greater refinement in outcome measurement so that these are more relevant to patients and practitioners, as current measures focus almost exclusively on impairment and physical function, with outcomes for carers being 'very rarely mentioned'. From a service perspective length of hospital stay is the most frequently adopted measure of success. Overall no study in the review utilized a full range of outcome measures covering the perception of service providers, older people and their carers.

This review raises a number of questions about the status presently accorded to the randomized controlled trial with its reliance on frequently superficial and often spurious indicators of success. It also further highlights the marked differences between the perceptions of professionals and those of disabled people, as noted in Chapter 1 in relation to quality of life.

The emphasis on outcome measurement is consistent with the notion that rehabilitation is a finite, time-limited process, with these two topics being given considerable prominence in the rehabilitation literature. A summary of this literature reinforces the conceptual limitations of most existing approaches to outcome measurement.

Although Swift (1996) contends that there are few universal indicators of outcome in rehabilitation, a meta-analysis carried out by Evans *et al.* (1995) concluded that outcomes are usually restricted to three broad areas: survival, functional ability and discharge destination. Indeed 'getting the patient home' is often the ultimate aim of rehabilitation (Waters 1991), and present economic concerns mean that a reduction in length of stay is likely to achieve ever greater prominence (Cope and Sundance 1995; Dejong and Sutton 1995; Keith 1995; Landrum *et al.* 1995). The appeal of outcomes which define an end-point, such as improved physical functioning, is therefore readily apparent.

Although outcomes such as survival and discharge destination provide clear-cut criteria, the need for further, more elaborate but still quantifiable indicators has resulted in considerable store being placed on scientific measurement in rehabilitation. Tallis (1989) forcibly argued that measurement is essential and others see functional scales as lying at the heart of rehabilitation (Studenski and Duncan 1993), with the production of 'Standardized Functional Assessment Measures' being the ultimate aim (Grainger *et al.* 1996). Such measures, it is argued, will identify which interventions work and how much input is required (Tallis 1989), so that specific therapies can be administered at a given point in time (Landrum *et al.* 1995).

If a physical orientation and measurement model has prominence in much of the medical literature, considerable disquiet is expressed by many authors. Some see nothing inherently wrong with measurement per se but bemoan the lack of a theoretical underpinning in rehabilitation and argue for something more than a simple empirical model (Beckmann and Ditlev 1992; Glueckauf *et al.* 1993; Keith and Lipsey 1993; McFall 1993; Keith 1995; Renwick and Friefild 1996). Conversely others see this measurement orientation as reductionist (Bach and Rioux 1996) and characteristic of a biomedical model where there is a 'test for every occasion' (Day and Jankey 1996).

Such concerns have led to calls for a wider conceptualization of rehabilitation in which quality of life represents the primary outcome (Bowling 1995b; Brown *et al.* 1996a; Fitzpatrick 1996; Renwick and Friefild 1996; Renwick *et al.* 1996). Furthermore, it is argued that outcome measures should reflect the perspective of the disabled person, rather than professionals (Bowling 1991; Schulz and Williamson 1993; Laman and Lankhorst 1994; Bowling 1995a; Mechanic 1995; Day and Jankey 1996).

Conversely there is also considerable debate about the validity and relevance of outcome measurement itself, as it suggests a finite input and a distinct end-point (Guthrie and Harvey 1994), allowing the specification of an 'ultimate desirable result' (Bryant 1995). Such an assumption ignores the fact that treatment and support, especially in chronic conditions, may be life-long (Keith and Lipsey 1993). Despite recent definitions stressing its finite nature it is now more widely recognized that rehabilitation should not relate just to the acute phase of an illness or disability (Palat 1992; Dejong and Sutton 1995) and that the goals of therapy must be consistent with the phase or stage of an illness or disability (Keith and Lipsey 1993; Cope and Sundance 1995; Brown *et al.* 1996a). This requires that both long-term and short-term goals are set, and that such goals are negotiated and agreed by all those involved (Andrews 1987; Thurgood 1990; Guthrie and Harvey 1994; Williams 1994).

Clearly a more informed debate about the role of outcome measurement is important as outcomes are seen as a 'key component' of all quality initiatives (Winyard 1995), representing the end-point of clinical effectiveness (Lakhani 1995). Certainly the potentially pernicious effects of a time-limited, outcome-driven model of rehabilitation on older people must be recognized if the current renewed policy emphasis is to be of maximum benefit.

Rehabilitation and older people

Perhaps one of the most telling accounts of the way in which rehabilitation discriminates against older, especially frail older, people was provided by Becker (1994) who, over a six-year period, charted the rehabilitation histories of 214 stroke patients. It emerged that staff identify two general categories of patients: 'rehabilitation candidates' and 'geriatric care'. The treatment these two groups received differed markedly and, according to Becker (1994), provides a clear indication of how ageism can be institutionalized in health care.

Becker (1994) concluded that rehabilitation is still based primarily on the ethic of contemporary medicine and the doctrine of cure, with functional independence being used by rehabilitation practitioners as a proxy for health. Consequently the potential to achieve functional independence was critical to being seen as a 'rehabilitation candidate'. De facto therefore 'good' candidates were almost invariably those who were younger and had suffered a less severe stroke. Patients lacking the attributes of 'good' candidates but who had been transferred to rehabilitation units were often infantalized and asked to perform what they perceived as meaningless tasks, without adequate explanation.

In marked contrast rehabilitation candidates received full explanations and staff advocated more vigorously on their behalf, creating an environment in which hope was fostered. The situation could not have been more different for persons who were designated as geriatric care patients who appeared to experience a continued withdrawal of hope without redirection to other goals.

The most invidious aspect was the relative powerlessness of patients, as their 'categorization' by professionals largely determined their future care options. On the basis of this study Becker (1994) concluded that the existing system of rehabilitation is 'exclusionary' and fosters age discrimination, suggesting that there is a need to rethink the entire basis of rehabilitation with older people in order to create legitimate goals for individuals with limited potential for functional improvement. Such goals would include contributing to a sense of well-being and fostering a sense of value and hope. Many of the elements of the senses outlined in Chapter 1 and elaborated further in the context of acute care by Davies *et al.* (1999) are apparent in Becker's suggestions.

Even the mainstream medical literature has expressed disquiet about the limitations of present models of rehabilitation when applied to older people. Ebrahim (1994), for example, noted that rehabilitation neglects the views of patients and, because of its emphasis on short-term outcomes, focuses on goals of questionable relevance. He argued that the challenge for measurement in rehabilitation is to look beyond survival, cure or recurrence as outcomes and to move towards a model which focuses on whether a patient's life accords with his or her wishes. This requires an approach which addresses the entire care career rather than prioritize certain outcomes at an arbitrary point in time (Ebrahim 1994).

J. Young (1996) has voiced similar sentiments, suggesting that 'the commonest incorrect assumption is that rehabilitation is time-limited, with a clear end point'. Criticizing the emphasis on physical functioning he went on to argue that rehabilitation should assist frail older individuals to realize their full potential, to resettle in the community and to find role fulfilment. Accordingly rehabilitation should comprise both 'hard' interventions aimed at physical aspects of care and 'soft' interventions which involve listening, understanding and counselling. Interestingly, although they derive from widely differing perspectives, there is a clear congruence between Young's suggestions and Irurito's (1996) concepts of 'firm hand' and 'soft hand' care noted earlier.

The therapy literature increasingly alludes to the importance of looking beyond physical functioning in order to consider whether activity has both purpose and meaning (Mayers 1995; Trombly 1995), with some arguing that one of the main aims of rehabilitation should be to instil a sense of hope (Spencer *et al.* 1997). Here the aim is to assist older people to create a vision for the future, to imagine possibilities and goals and to sustain a positive sense of direction in the face of major losses.

The importance of active family involvement in rehabilitation is also increasingly acknowledged in the literature, although families are often expected to accept the decisions of professionals passively, and thereby remain marginal figures in the rehabilitation process (McColl 1995). Clark *et al.* (1994) for example argue that occupational therapists (OTs) often fail to develop a therapeutic relationship with family carers, frequently seeing them as a hindrance rather than a help. Consequently, most interventions focus on technical issues and the goals of therapy, with far less attention being given to actively involving carers.

In the context of the 'carers as experts' model described in Chapter 2, rehabilitation is a critical period in which family members have to make informed decisions about whether to care or not and, for those who decide to care, to learn the skills necessary. Unfortunately this opportunity is rarely realized, with little attention being given to the way that carers 'take on' their role (Given and Given 1991; Nolan and Grant 1992a; Stewart *et al.* 1993). Consequently studies suggest that carers often do not exercise genuine choice (Taraborrelli 1993), and are frequently unaware of the extent and nature of their caring responsibilities (Allen *et al.* 1983; Lewis and Meredith 1988a, b; Nolan and Grant 1992a). There is little professional input at this time and carers are rarely fully prepared, either physically or psychologically, for their role, frequently lacking the necessary knowledge and skills (Braithwaite 1990; Kemp 1993; Stewart *et al.* 1993; Harvath *et al.* 1994; Lea 1994). Subsequently carers acquire knowledge and skills largely by a process of trial and error, a situation which has been described as 'flailing about' (Stewart *et al.* 1993). During this period carers have a particular need for information which is often not met (Strauss *et al.* 1984; Thorne 1993) and they are usually at the 'bottom of the institutional hierarchy of information' (Strauss *et al.* 1984). If the needs of carers are assessed at all they are often 'tacked on' at the end of the rehabilitation process (Bowles *et al.* 1995) reinforcing the suggestion of Waters and Luker (1996) that carers do not figure prominently.

The above conclusions are further supported by Brereton and Nolan (2000) in a qualitative study exploring the way in which carers of individuals who have had a stroke are prepared for their role. Based on an analysis of data from the experiences of carers during hospitalization until shortly after discharge, four key themes emerged:

'What's it all about'	capturing carers' lack of understanding of stroke and the difficulties they had in obtaining a comprehensive but appropriate explanation
'Going it alone'	reflecting carers' exasperation with the formal care system and their consequent reliance on their own, often limited, resources
'Up to the job'	describing the struggle that carers experienced to gain the knowledge and skills they needed to feel competent to provide the care required
'What about me'	highlighting the lack of attention both to carers' needs and to the biographical knowledge they had of the person with stroke.

Although small scale, this study provides a telling account of how little attention is given to carers who were expected to care for heavily dependent individuals, with little or no real support.

Moreover, despite the introduction of the Carers Act, which affords a statutory right of assessment to carers 'providing or intending to provide care', other, more extensive, recent studies suggest that carers' situation has not improved. Poor discharge arrangements are still prevalent, with carers lacking information and support, with their comments often being ignored (Henwood 1998; Warner and Wexler 1998). Therefore while discharge represents an ideal opportunity to help and advise carers, only 38 per cent feel that their needs are assessed, 40 per cent feel unprepared at discharge, with 70 per cent not having had the opportunity to discuss alternative care options and 71 per cent not receiving a copy of a discharge plan (Henwood 1998). Similarly Warner and Wexler (1998) found that carers were seldom consulted, rarely trained and only occasionally asked if they could cope. Although these surveys used non-random samples, they represent the experiences of several hundred carers drawn from disparate sources and provide a telling indication of the limitations of current models of assessing carers' needs. Clearly there is a need for a considerable reorientation of current practice if even the modest aims of the Carers' National Strategy are to be achieved.

Advancing rehabilitation

If the recent emphasis on rehabilitation is to lead to improved services for older people, there is a need for a more holistic orientation which acknowledges a diversity of outcomes and approaches. Issues relating to outcomes are of particular significance in the context of older people. On the one hand there are calls to develop a standardized approach with a 'comprehensive geriatric assessment' seen as the key to quality and effectiveness (Carpenter and Calnan 1997), but on the other hand it is argued that current outcomes are based on an overly simplistic model which fails to capture the diversity and complexity of need in older people (Ebrahim *et al.* 1993). Further fuelling this debate, Evans (1997) has argued that the specification of appropriate and sensitive outcome measures for older people represents one of the greatest challenges for the future. He contends that the use of 'collectivist' measures based on the life review of the 'average citizen' are largely irrelevant to most older people as they fail to account for the heterogeneity within this population. Instead he advocates the development of individual indices of quality of life to identify the objectives for care and to evaluate the success of interventions.

Rehabilitation still focuses almost exclusively on physical functioning, however; even those instruments with a more expansive conceptual basis, such as quality of life indicators, usually reflect the normative judgements of professionals. Outcomes, it seems, are increasingly driven by cost considerations and professional ideologies so that they are often irrelevant to the everyday lives of disabled people (Stover 1995), overlooking individual narratives in favour of standardized models (Spencer *et al.* 1995), thereby negating the 'existential experience' of chronic illness and disability (Quinn *et al.* 1995). This, as Nolan *et al.* (1997) argue, is characteristic of the 'restricted isolated model' rather than a more relevant comprehensive integrative approach.

Others too recognize the limitations of rehabilitation practice and some years ago Ory and Williams (1989) called for a new approach to rehabilitation with older people underpinned by five principles:

- The setting of small goals in order that regular progress can be made.
- Life-course timing – a consideration of what the disability means and what the person brings to the rehabilitation encounter.
- An understanding of the disability as perceived by all the parties involved.
- Fostering social support and providing help for family carers.
- Full recognition of the long duration of rehabilitation, which is often a life-long process, particularly in the case of disability which is progressive or uncertain.

Working from similar premises, although not referring exclusively to older people, Pawlson (1994) advocated a 'new paradigm' of health care more relevant to the needs of modern society. In so doing he contrasted what he termed the 'Simple Acute Disease Model' with a 'Complex Chronic Illness Model', which viewed the patient as an active participant in rehabilitation rather than a passive recipient. While Pawlson (1994) viewed this approach as more appropriate a simple acute model still dominates.

Barolin (1996) also proposed a new model of rehabilitation for older people which moves beyond physical functioning, recognizes that rehabilitation is not a finite process and does not see advanced age as a barrier. The aim of such an approach is to improve overall quality of life, with rehabilitation taking place across care environments and contexts. This provides particular challenges in a community setting, which forms the substance of Chapter 4.

The literature on the needs of older people in acute care and rehabilitative settings is diverse and emanates from several professional disciplines, as well as differing theoretical orientations. Consistent with the aims of this book, the main focus in this chapter has been on the needs of frail older people and their carers, with an emphasis on comparing potentially contrasting perceptions of the purposes of care and how these may impact on quality of life.

Mirroring the themes emerging from the 'scene-setting' Chapters 1 and 2, it is apparent that the way services are perceived by professionals and older people or carers often differ markedly. In acute care in particular there is growing recognition of the need to combine competent technical care with excellent interpersonal care, with skills in both these areas being required by practitioners. For this to be achieved interpersonal elements have to be accorded greater value and status. Furthermore, given the complexity of need in older people assessment is increasingly recognized as a key component of the care process, but there are searching questions being asked about the quality of current practice and the skills and knowledge of practitioners in a number of areas. The literature on rehabilitation further highlights the way in which professionally defined services and their outcomes can be at variance with the aspirations of older people and their carers, a tension that will be further explored in Chapter 4, which considers primary and community care.

4

Community care

Janet Nolan

A major contemporary social goal is to keep even frail older people in their community home. It is thus essential to identify what kinds of enrichments or services might be needed to elevate quality of life for elders so disabled as to require continuing in-home care.

(Lawton *et al.* 1995: 151)

The influence of older people on the design of outcome measures or the specification of relevant domains appears minimal. Most measures reflect normative professional judgements about areas which are important influences on the likelihood of continuing at home, rather than those factors which have been identified as contributing to quality of life.

(Nocon and Qureshi 1996: 88)

The initial chapters in this book have highlighted a number of themes which inform current debates about how services can maintain or improve the quality of care and the quality of life of older people. Many of these reflect implicit or explicit tensions along a number of dimensions, including the following:

- Economic considerations about reducing or controlling costs which potentially conflict with humanitarian principles concerned with maintaining individuality and ensuring equity of access.
- The focus on objective measures of outcome which identify clearly specified end-points as opposed to subjective and perceptual dimensions which capture individual aspirations.
- Professional definitions of service objectives which often contrast with those of older people and their carers.

Such considerations are brought into particularly sharp relief when community care for older people is considered. As noted in Chapter 1, globally, the main aim of policy for older people is to maintain the individual in their chosen environment, which is widely recognized as being their own home. However, as the above quotations suggest, this raises difficult questions about how quality of life can be promoted, particularly for frail older people.

The purpose of this chapter is to explore further a number of dilemmas relating to community care for older people and to consider their implications for the design, delivery and evaluation of services and for professional practice and education. The chapter begins with a brief overview of community care as it relates to older people and their carers, with attention subsequently being turned to an analysis of three areas which are illustrative of a range of potentially contradictory influences. These are preventive and rehabilitative services, meeting the needs of frail older people and addressing carers' needs.

Community care and older people

There can be few policy objectives which have been the subject of such detailed analysis as community care. Despite this, Kane (1999) suggests that surprisingly little thought has been given to the intended outcomes for older people, other than to maintain the individual at home. As Henwood (1992) noted, searching questions need to be asked about the objectives of community care in order to avoid initiatives being a 'leap in the dark'. A similar plea was made by Walker (1995b), who called for a new vision of community care based on clear policy goals. Walker (1995b) believes that notwithstanding 'half a century of promises', current policy continues to fail older people with the views of service providers and professionals still dominating, as agencies actively compete to shed responsibility for service provision to the most frail and vulnerable older people.

A number of other commentators suggest that despite persuasive humanitarian arguments in favour of community care, underlying motives are primarily economic, to do with minimizing costs by preventing admission to hospital or residential care, and facilitating rapid discharge from expensive acute care facilities (Wistow 1995; Hanford *et al.* 1999). Moreover, despite the taken-for-granted superiority of living at home (Baldwin *et al.* 1993), the notion that community services can provide a viable alternative to institutional care has not been rigorously tested (Henwood 1992) and Dalley (1998) maintains that the efficacy of community care remains largely an 'article of faith'.

In their detailed analysis of the emergence of community care policy, Nocon and Qureshi (1996) attribute current objectives largely to the White Paper *Caring for People* (Department of Health 1989a), suggesting that this promoted three central aims, these being to

- enable people to live as normal a life as possible in their own homes or in a homely environment in the community
- provide the right amount of care and support to help people achieve maximum independence and, by acquiring or reacquiring basic living skills, help them to achieve their full potential
- give people a greater individual say in how they live their lives and in the design of services.

The influence of these themes remains evident in contemporary initiatives, such as pervasive notions of empowerment and partnership (Ogg *et al.* 1998; Malin *et al.* 1999), and in the drive towards promoting independence which figures so prominently in recent policy statements and service priorities for both the health and social services (Department of Health 1998b, c).

As Nocon and Qureshi (1996) note, the concept of a 'normal life' is a relative one and the identification of clear objectives has been inhibited by our limited understanding of what older people expect from community care or the type of 'normal life' to which they aspire. This is manifestly the case in relation to frail older people, as there has been little theoretical or empirical work considering the views and perceptions of those in receipt of care, whether from formal services or family carers (Lawton *et al.* 1995; Cox and Dooley 1996; Seale 1996; Twigg 1998). Greater clarity will remain elusive until we move beyond the language of 'general principles' (Henwood 1992) and can specify with more precision the aims and objectives of community care for older people.

Table 4.1 provides a synthesis of some recent reflections on the aims of community care for older people, at both policy and service delivery levels. While these are still couched largely as general principles, there is an emergent consensus with moves towards greater specificity being apparent, especially in Kane's (1999) analysis. The objectives identified by Nocon and Qureshi (1996) followed an extensive consideration of the then available literature, and the recent work by Easterbrook (1999) and Farell *et al.* (1999) is particularly illuminating, being the result of new empirical studies with older people, family carers and service providers.

Farell *et al.* (1999) based their conclusions on focus group interviews with older and disabled people and their carers, exploring their experiences of health, housing and social services and staff providing treatment and care. In contrast Easterbrook (1999) synthesized the views of service providers about how care for older people could be improved. Promisingly, there is considerable congruence between these two studies suggesting that, in principle at least, staff are sensitive to the needs of older people and acknowledge that services should be flexible, individualized and of high quality, provided by staff with the appropriate skills and competencies.

Continuity of staff and confidence in their ability to deliver often complex care packages were seen as being particularly important (Farell *et al.*

Table 4.1 Community care: aims and aspirations

Policy		Services			
Provide for ethnic diversity Combat ageist practice Recognize diversity of lifestyle Facilitate greater involvement Value elders as resources (Evandrou, 1998)	The adoption of intergenerational life-course perspective with a focus on 'Ageing not old age' Policy based on a pluralistic, preventive, positive view of ageing Combat all forms of discrimination Empowerment Citizenship rights Hearing the voices of ordinary people The need for both critical commentary and action (Bernard and Phillips 1998)	Respect as a fellow human being Autonomy about life's decisions Treat as an individual Recognize totality of need Choice Recognizing carers' needs Partnership (Nocon and Qureshi 1996)	Maintain dignity Provide real choice Foster autonomy Treat as partner Allow to live an ordinary life involving: Participation Rewarding activity Maintaining relationships (Easterbrook 1999)	Honesty Positive approach Partnership Equality/freedom of choice To be treated with respect To be listened to (Farell et al. 1999)	To improve/maintain health Promote comfort/freedom from pain Improve/show deterioration in function Meet needs for assistance/care Improve knowledge/self-help abilities Enhance psychological well-being Enhance social well-being Promote a meaningful life Maximize independence/autonomy Allow to be at home (Kane 1999)

1999) but unfortunately older people often felt that staff were poorly prepared to meet their needs and demonstrated discriminatory, patronizing
and demeaning attitudes. To compound such difficulties, access to services
was frequently inhibited by poor assessment procedures, with eligibility criteria being incomprehensible to many older people (Farell *et al.* 1999). These
authors called for a 'distinctive cultural shift' among service providers,
requiring greater recognition of the principles identified in Table 4.1. Others
have also argued for a reorientation of practice so that services enhance the
skills, independence and decision-making capacity of individuals (Malin *et
al.* 1999) and move away from a culture of dependency (Phillipson and
Biggs 1998) towards a model which recognizes the assets older people have
and not just their deficits (Kivnick and Murray 1997; Evandrou 1998).

Easterbrook's (1999) study suggests that practitioners involved in front-
line care delivery for older people are highly critical of current services and
bemoan the lack of a coherent vision for community care. These practitioners endorsed the principles summarized in Table 4.1, and argued that
staff should be able to work across agency boundaries and recognize that
this requires training that places greater emphasis on social and interpersonal skills (Easterbrook 1999). Additionally, one of the major concerns
to emerge from this study was the low status of both older people and the
staff who support them. This situation is unlikely to improve until the
skills and competencies required to work with older people are not only
better understood, but also valued and promoted. This is an issue that will
be returned to later.

Kane's (1999) analysis, although developed in the context of the US
system, has wider relevance particularly in the light of recent White Papers
and subsequent advisory documents (Department of Health 1997a, 1998a,
b, c) which place considerable emphasis on improving quality so that services reflect the experiences of users and carers. Debates about the intended
outcomes of care are particularly prominent in relation to social services
(Department of Health 1998b, c) and Kane (1999) provides a useful conceptualization of what the aims of community care for older people could
or should be. However, she notes that although policy makers subscribe to
such goals in principle, the more diffuse elements such as the enhancement of well-being and the promotion of a meaningful life are rarely
explicitly resourced and consequently remain largely at the level of
rhetoric. Indeed Kane's framework reflects many of the tensions identified
throughout this book and these will now be explored further in relation to
preventive and rehabilitative services for older people.

Preventive and rehabilitative care: the new panacea?

The promotion of independence is one of the government's key policy
objectives for both the health and social services (Department of Health

1997a). Consequently, in addition to the current emphasis on rehabilitation highlighted in Chapter 3, there has been an increasing focus on preventive care. One concrete manifestation of this is the introduction of
prevention grants intended to signal a new era of collaboration between
service agencies, facilitating the development of low level support services
which enable more older people to remain at home in the hope of reducing admission to hospital and care homes (Hanford *et al.* 1999). The
impact of this initiative for those individuals currently receiving more
intensive packages of care has yet to be determined, however, but is potentially significant given the increased levels of frailty among many older
people now being supported in the community (Audit Commission 1999).
This is explored further in the section that follows.

The onus now being placed on preventive services provides an elegant
case example which highlights many of the tensions which emerge when
such concepts are applied to older people. At a theoretical level, Wetle
(1998) suggests that research into reducing disability and increasing
healthy lifespan constitute two of the most significant challenges for
gerontological research beyond the year 2000. He highlights in particular
the need to explore patterns of disability among older people so as better
to understand how to promote health by attention to lifestyle factors such
as a low fat, high fibre diet; exercise; giving up smoking; moderating alcohol and medication use; and preventive services such as screening and
early diagnosis. His arguments mirror the considerable recent interest in
the compression of morbidity among older people, in order to enable
them to live as much of their lives as possible free from disability (Mathers and Robine 1998; Prophet 1998). Mathers and Robine (1998), in
reviewing the international evidence, suggest that although results are as
yet equivocal there is some indication that disability levels are falling
slightly, but that paradoxically this does not seem to be accompanied by
improvements in subjective well-being.

Prophet (1998), in marshalling evidence to present to the Royal Commission on Long-Term Care on behalf of the Continuing Care Conference,
provides a strong economic case for compressing morbidity, arguing that
a fall in morbidity among older people of 1 per cent per annum would, by
2030, result in a 30 per cent reduction in welfare costs, amounting to an
annual saving of some £6.5 billion. Consequently the Continuing Care
Conference strongly recommends that compression of morbidity should
be an explicit policy objective, requiring the development of preventive
and rehabilitative services, augmented by awareness-raising campaigns in
a number of areas, such as promoting exercise and reducing hypertension,
smoking and alcohol intake. They also advocate greater use of disability-
delaying technologies in conditions such as incontinence, hip and knee
surgery and cataracts. In promoting these arguments it was suggested that
two general types of service should be developed, one to prevent or delay
ill-health and disability and the other to improve quality of life and
engagement in the community. Such initiatives are seen as essential if the

legitimate aspirations of older people are to be met. Such aspirations, according to Prophet (1998), are similar to those of adults of all ages and include

- being seen as an individual
- having a range of friendships and relationships
- feeling independent
- feeling safe
- being as healthy as possible
- feeling in control of life
- focusing on what people can do as well as the difficulties they face.

Similarly, in its analysis of the responses of local authorities to the current preventive agenda, the Joseph Rowntree Foundation (1999) identified two broad approaches, these being:

- strategies that prevent or delay the need for more costly services
- strategies to maintain and improve quality of life.

When exploring service developments, the foundation discovered considerable variation across England, concluding that if preventive strategies are to be successfully introduced, there is a need both to combat ageist attitudes and to be creative in the use of resources (Joseph Rowntree Foundation 1999). This requires a more informed debate about the intended benefits of preventive care. This is essential because agencies which are currently under pressure to demonstrate results focus mainly on quantifiable indicators of success such as reduced expenditure and give a very limited consideration to subjective dimensions of quality of life. Unless this trend is countered, priority will continue to be given to strategies designed to reduce the need for costly services rather than those promoting quality of life. This reinforces Kane's (1999) contention that despite the rhetoric of holistic outcomes there are factors operating within service systems which conspire to ensure that objective measures of success are more highly valued.

The Joseph Rowntree Foundation (1999) argues that if a preventive culture is to flourish then a number of structures have to be developed including

- cross-agency and cross-sector commitment
- engaging older people in service design and delivery
- locally based initiatives
- institutional commitment at a senior level
- dedicated budgets and staff.

Success will remain elusive unless ageist attitudes that perpetuate the belief that older people have neither the desire nor the capacity to participate fully in their care can be countered. Such attitudes are very evident in the literature on health promotion.

It is widely recognized that the main goals of health promotion with older people are to maintain independence (Richmond and McCracken 1996; Dahlin-Ivanoff *et al.* 1998; Minkler and Checkoway 1998), delay dependency and disability (While 1990; Conn and Armer 1996) and improve quality of life (While 1990), but these aims are rarely realized. Despite the expansion of the literature on health promotion, very little of this focuses on older people (Gillis and Hirdes 1996), who are often excluded from research studies (Lauder 1993; Victor and Higginson 1994). There is consequently a dearth of empirical evidence on the effectiveness of health promotion programmes with older people. Greengross *et al.* (1997) argue that older people have often been patronized or 'neglected' by the health promotion movement (Bettison 1988), with their needs being given a low priority. Ageist assumptions about the limited benefits of promoting the health of older people (Victor and Higginson 1994) have resulted in a poor understanding of their health status and the factors that might influence it (Greengross *et al.* 1997; Poxton 1998). Frequently the results of studies focusing on younger age groups are extrapolated to older people (Uitenbroek 1996) a strategy which is of questionable value (Gillis and Hirdes 1996). Furthermore, despite the plethora of recent policy pronouncements relating to health promotion, many of these ignored or gave limited attention to the needs of older people (K. Young 1996; Dalley 1998; Peate 1999).

Despite this unsatisfactory situation, there has been growing interest in the possible benefits to older people of lifestyle changes including:

- exercise and physical activity (Conn and Armer 1996; Travis *et al.* 1996; Allison and Keller 1997)
- giving up smoking (Greengross *et al.* 1997; Khaw 1997; Prophet 1998; Wetle 1998)
- better diet (Prophet 1998; Wetle 1998)
- reducing alcohol consumption (Herring and Thom 1997; Prophet 1998; Wetle 1998)

Programmes targeted at these areas have a number of potential benefits, including reducing the incidence of coronary heart disease, strokes, osteoporosis and cancer among others. There is also scope for promoting better mental health among older people, an issue which forms the substance of Chapter 7. While health promotion with older people offers considerable promise, the impact of new threats to health such as stress, pollution and food contamination also need to be considered (Evandrou 1998).

Another pressing issue is who will deliver a health promotion agenda with older people. A major thematic review on services for older people (Audit Commission 1997), supported by much of the literature, concluded that this is a role that could be fulfilled by community nurses, particularly district nurses and health visitors (see Table 4.2). Despite this there are formidable barriers, both attitudinal and organizational, that inhibit practitioners from realizing such potential roles (see Table 4.3).

Moreover, although potentially significant, preventive measures in

Table 4.2 Health promotion and older people: potential roles for community nurses

---

Undertaking holistic health assessment
Machell *et al.* 1988; Alford and Futrell 1992; Peate 1999

Considering wider issues affecting health such as transport and accessibility
Kaplan *et al.* 1987; Harber 1989; Alford and Futrell 1992; Department of Health 1995c

Promoting comprehensive screening
Powell and Crombie 1974; Charmove and Young 1989; Dahlin-Ivanoff *et al.* 1998

Improving health through empowerment
Ide and Wolff 1993; Beckingham and Watt 1995

Improving health through education
Williamson 1988; Janes 1993; Marr 1994; Allison and Keller 1997

Encouraging self-care
Kart and Dunkle 1989; Beckingham and Watt 1995

Recognizing the older person's ability to enhance their own health
Alford and Futrell 1992; Frenn 1996; J. Young 1996

Using health promotion strategies that are acceptable and relevant to older people
Cirincoine and Fattore 1996

---

isolation are unlikely to be optimally effective and if the expectations of older people to have a healthy and active retirement are to be realized, a range of other factors such as housing, income and harnessing technology also have to be considered (Alford and Futrell 1992; J. Young 1996; Evandrou 1998). In promoting this broader conceptualization of what constitutes preventive interventions, Prophet (1998) cites the work of Wistow and Lewis (1997), who outline a number of strategies aimed at:

- delaying or reducing the impact of biological processes
- minimizing socio-economic differences
- helping older people build social networks in the community
- informing attitudes and expectations of older people
- addressing environmental factors.

Environmental factors are particularly important in enabling frail older people to remain in their own homes and the wider application of technology for both frail older people and their carers is considered in more detail shortly.

Developing in tandem with the preventive agenda, and some might argue

Table 4.3 Health promotion and older people: barriers to community nurses playing a fuller role

---

Focusing primarily on disease rather than being holistic in their approach
Bergen and La Bute 1993; Ide and Wolff 1993; Stokes 1994

Seeing themselves rather than older people as experts
Beckingham and Watt 1995

Consequently underestimating the health potential of older people
Beckingham and Watt 1995

Undervaluing health promotion work with older people
Bettison 1988; Alford and Futrell 1992; Lauder 1993; Pursey and Luker 1993; Hardman *et al.* 1995

Neglecting their potential role in health promotion
Burridge 1988; Machell *et al.* 1988; Marr 1994; Victor and Higginson 1994

Displaying ageist attitudes
Machell *et al.* 1988; Victor 1991; Lauder 1993; Pursey and Luker 1993; Victor and Higginson 1994; Murphy and Hepworth 1996; Peate 1999

Feeling ill equipped to take on health promotion role
Turton and Faulkner 1983; Phillipson and Strang 1985; While 1990

Feeling unable to undertake role because of increased work loads
Phillipson and Strang 1985

Decreasing staffing levels
Phillipson and Strang 1985

According other work priority
Burridge 1988; While 1990

Lacking time
Burridge 1988

---

subsumed within it, are moves to extend rehabilitation to a community setting (Nocon and Baldwin 1998; Sinclair and Dickinson 1998). As noted in Chapter 3, rehabilitation provides a paradigm case highlighting a number of tensions which have to be addressed if notions of empowerment and partnership are to be realized. Such tensions are reflected in the contrasting 'restricted isolated' and 'comprehensive integrative' models of rehabilitation outlined by Nolan *et al.* (1997) and are brought into even sharper relief when the rehabilitation needs of older people in a community context are considered.

Rehabilitation in a community context

According to Prophet (1998) the goals of rehabilitation are to facilitate early hospital discharge, reduce long-term care placement and increase the cost-effective use of resources, while simultaneously promoting quality of life. These reflect the potentially contradictory aims of community care identified by Kane (1999) and as the recent work on the implementation of preventive strategies indicates (Joseph Rowntree Foundation 1999), the outcomes of rehabilitation are likely to continue to be judged primarily by objective measures. Furthermore, despite the rhetoric of services reflecting the experiences and aspirations of older people and their carers (Department of Health 1998a, b, c), current definitions of rehabilitation are still based primarily on a restorative model (Nocon and Baldwin 1998). Such an orientation does not necessarily provide a 'comfortable fit' in a community context, where continuity of care and being able to 'engage with life' are equally important considerations (Hasselkus *et al.* 1997). Therefore, while enabling an older person to return home is a legitimate goal, it is of limited value unless accompanied by a sense of identity, security, order and control (Hasselkus *et al.* 1997).

It is this contrast between objective and easily quantifiable measures of rehabilitation and the more subtle, diffuse, biographical and existential concerns of disabled people that highlights the importance of an holistic approach (Nolan *et al.* 1997), a point emphasized some time ago by Robinson (1988) as illustrated in Table 4.4.

Table 4.4 Contrasting rehabilitation models

Short-term rehabilitation model	*Long-term rehabilitation model*
Focus on impairment or disability	Focus on handicap
Technique orientated	Patient orientated
Doctor as controller	Doctor as coordinator
Therapist as agent	Therapist as autonomous
Hospital based	Community based

Source: After Robinson 1988

It is clear that promoting rehabilitation in a community context has a number of implications for the way in which outcomes are conceptualized and that a finite, time-limited model has limited relevance. Others also promote a temporal dimension with, for example, Cope and Sundance (1995) identifying six phases or stages in the rehabilitation process:

- physiologic instability
- physiologic stability
- physiologic maintenance
- residential integration

- community reintegration
- productive activity.

Cope and Sundance (1995) argue that traditional approaches to rehabilitation focus predominantly on attaining physiologic maintenance, with the aim of returning people home. Subsequently however, little attention is given to residential integration and even less to community reintegration and productive activity. Other models of rehabilitation also promote a more holistic focus as illustrated by Nolan *et al.* (1997), who used the International Classification of Impairment, Disability and Handicap (World Health Organisation 1980) as an heuristic device and summarized a number of approaches to rehabilitation (see Table 4.5).

As can be seen, such frameworks suggest that rehabilitation should input at a number of levels including primary, secondary and tertiary interventions. These models would probably be rejected by Nocon and Baldwin (1998) as they fail to meet the criterion of differentiating rehabilitation from other services. However, such a criterion is largely created and sustained by service and agency ideologies in order that respective responsibilities can be clearly delineated, but, if the intention is to ensure that responses to users' needs do not simply reflect current service boundaries (Department of Health 1998b), then differentiating rehabilitation, as advocated by Nocon and Baldwin (1998) seems a rather fruitless pursuit. This is unlikely to facilitate continuity of care which is so important to older people and their carers (Banks 1999; Farell *et al.* 1999).

While policy promotes rehabilitation in community settings, practice still focuses mainly on the early stages of the disablement process, with interventions being targeted mostly on improving functional ability. The onus is therefore largely on rehabilitation within hospital settings, yet the majority of the care and rehabilitation occur within the community where the greatest deficits in service provision exist (Beardshaw 1988; Barker *et al.* 1997). For example an extensive review by Lafferty (1996) suggested that the transfer of rehabilitation from hospital to the community is consistent with a number of policy objectives and assumes a range of benefits including

- the patient's natural desire to return home
- reduction of hospitalization
- better assessment of rehabilitation potential at home
- cost savings.

Despite such putative benefits, Lafferty (1996) argued that there is little evidence of the effectiveness of rehabilitation in the patient's home, as existing studies pay scant attention to the social, psychological and financial costs to patients and carers. While Philp (1996) supports community rehabilitation in principle, he cautions that it must not become community neglect, advocating that the effectiveness of community alternatives should be established before the existing hospital infrastructure is dismantled.

Table 4.5 Different conceptualization of rehabilitation

Model	Level	Stage	Purpose	Responsibility/focus
Livneh 1995 Tripartite model	Predisease Impairment Disability Handicap	Primary Secondary (crisis) Tertiary (I) Tertiary (II) Tertiary (III)	Reduce/prevent disability Preserve life Minimize disability Compensate for disability Modify environment	Acute medical interventions OT, physio, speech Therapist, counselling, social work Vocational rehabilitation
Hershenson 1990	Predisease Impairment Disability Handicap	Primary Secondary ⟷ Tertiary	Reduce/prevent disability Reduce functional limitations Prevent limitations becoming handicaps	Public health (environment) Medicine, therapy (person) Rehabilitation counselling (person and environment)
Hunt 1980 (cited by Andrews 1987) SPREAD model	Predisease Impairment Disability Handicap		Specific control of disease Prevention of secondary disability Restorative measure Adaptation	Medical Nursing/therapy Therapy/nursing Therapy/social work
Cope and Sundance 1995	Predisease Impairment Disability Handicap	Physiologic instability Physiologic stability Physiologic maintenance Residual reintegration Community reintegration Productive activity	Preserve life Prevent complications to skin, etc. Environment of choice Community of choice Recreation, social activity relevant to life stages and interests	Medicine/intensive nursing Nursing Therapy

Source: Nolan *et al.* 1997

It is clear that if rehabilitation in the community is to develop then more thought has to be given to professional roles and methods of working. For example, in their extensive analysis of the nursing literature on rehabilitation Nolan *et al.* (1997) identified a diverse number of potential roles, as illustrated in Table 4.6.

Just as with health promotion, such roles are rarely fully developed, as practitioners often lack the necessary knowledge and skills, a deficit that has numerous implications for the education and training of professionals.

One of the most significant challenges to the development of both preventive and rehabilitation services, and community care more generally, is how to meet the needs of frail older people and their carers. Indeed if the much vaunted but still elusive quest to enhance quality of life for older people is to be addressed, then the needs of frail older people require a more comprehensive consideration.

Frail older people: the conundrum of community care?

In addition to promoting independence, one of the principal aims of current policy is to ensure that people live a 'meaningful' life (Department of Health 1998b). What constitutes a meaningful life is likely to be the subject of considerable individual variation, particularly for those agencies providing services to frail older people living in the community.

As Kane (1999) suggested, while most policy makers generally endorse the need to sustain a meaningful life, there is only a limited appreciation of what this means and often even less financial commitment. However, for Kane (1999) the issue is an important one as she believes that unacceptable numbers of older people in the community experience a life 'not worth living'. Other commentators also highlight the importance of older people being able to engage in a 'meaningful personal project' (Seale 1996) and have questioned how services might assist them in achieving such an aim (Lawton *et al.* 1995). As was noted in Chapter 1, opinions are very divergent, with some commentators promoting notions of autonomy and independence while others point to the growing body of evidence suggesting that an understanding of what constitutes a 'successful life' in older age must take full account of the importance of interdependent relationships. Paradoxically while self-reliance is often 'lionized' (Kivnick and Murray 1997) this may serve only to heighten a sense of dependence among very frail older people (Minkler 1996).

The type of 'shrunken world' that frail older people living in the community can occupy was captured by Lawton *et al.* (1995). Employing a 'yesterday interview', in which family carers described the previous 24 hours, they revealed that older people were passive for over 80 per cent of their time, with only 7 per cent being spent in 'enriching activities' compared

Table 4.6 Some suggested components of the nursing role in rehabilitation and chronic illness

Waters 1987	Corbin and Strauss 1991	Hymovich and Hagopian 1992	Brillhart and Sills 1994	Lamb and Stempel 1994	Hoeman 1996
Risk taker	Direct care	Establish/maintain trust	Caregiver	Technical expert	Educator
Enabler	Teach	Provide support/guidance	Counsellor	Monitoring	Counsellor
Healer	Counsel	Provide information	Collaborator	Coordinating	Care manager
Achiever	Make referrals	Provide anticipatory guidance	Educator	Teaching	Researcher
Befriender	Make arrangements	Facilitate stress reduction	Communicator	Enabling	Advocate
Imagination (user of)	Monitor	Facilitate self-care	Manager		Enabler and
facilitator					
Love (giver of moderated)		Facilitate access to resources	Staff developer		Teacher
Independence (facilitator of)		Modify attitudes			Expert practitioner
Treatment (giver of)		Assess all family members			Team member
		Provide direct care			
Adviser		Collaborate with others			
Teacher					
Intimate care (giver of)					
Organizer					
Nurturer					

with approximately 23 per cent for a similarly aged but less frail cohort. Only 3 out of 116 older people had been involved in any recreational activity on the day of the study and the authors therefore queried whether their quality of life was acceptable. While they recognized the existence of strong personal preferences for remaining at home, Lawton *et al.* (1995) challenged the accepted wisdom that a home environment is necessarily more stimulating than one within a care home. Baldwin *et al.* (1993) noted similar concerns and questioned the taken-for-granted superiority of living at home noting:

> Many older people at home cope without the benefit of regular care. In such circumstances depersonalisation, loneliness, withdrawal and depression may be common and might in other contexts be described as institutionalisation.
>
> (Baldwin *et al.* 1993: 757)

Clearly therefore the aims of community care must extend beyond keeping older people at home and preventing placement (Clark 1995; Kane 1999) and should include a consideration of the sorts of 'enrichments' that can be provided (Lawton *et al.* 1995) in order to promote meaningful involvement and engagement (Clark 1995; Seale 1996; Johnson and Barer 1997; Kane 1999). The paucity of empirical studies focusing on the experiences of elderly care-receivers (Cartwright *et al.* 1994; Lawton *et al.* 1995; Nolan *et al.* 1996a; Seale 1996) reinforces the need for further work in this area but the limited available evidence suggests the potential for interventions on a number of fronts.

Lawton *et al.* (1995) for example stress the importance of providing sensory, cognitive and social challenges, arguing that this should be seen as essentially therapeutic rather than simply diversional. They extol the potential role of technology in broadening the horizons for older people by increasing their sense of control and empowering them to make choices, as well as providing avenues for wider social contact. Others also see technology as empowering (Bernard and Phillips 1998; Evandrou 1998; Prophet 1998) advocating the wider application and fuller development of concepts such as the 'Lifetime home' or the 'Smart home' in providing safer, more efficient and less dependency creating environments. Recent studies have taken a novel approach to the application of technology by harnessing the power of personal computers, CD-Rom and ISDN lines in providing older people and their carers with both direct, live, visual links with a health centre and interactive information on a range of topics such as coping in emergency situations, financial advice and social security benefits available and choosing respite care or a care home (Hanson and Clarke 2000; Hanson *et al.* 2000). While still at the developmental stage, early results are encouraging but highlight the need to overcome fears about the use of technology, limit its potential for the invasion of privacy and the importance of providing information at an early stage in the caregiving/care-receiving trajectory. As Bernard and Phillips (1998) suggest, the potential applications of technology are extensive and this is one area in which the quality of life for frail older people could be significantly improved.

Another area which would benefit from further conceptual and empirical development is a fuller understanding of the nature and quality of interdependent relationships between older people and those providing support, whether family or formal carers. At the start of the 1990s Kahana and Young (1990) were critical of the existing simplistic models of caring relationships, arguing for the development of a more sophisticated approach that more fully reflected the dynamic, interactive and contextual nature of relationships as they evolved over time. Their vision was of an expanded caregiving paradigm that extended beyond dyadic relationships and incorporated the often delicate interactions between older people, family and formal caring systems. Unfortunately, the intervening decade has seen disappointingly little work in this area.

Some new insights have emerged with potential implications for the design and delivery of support. Seale (1996) for instance suggests that the central dilemma for carers is how to provide support in a way that sustains, rather that undermines, the care-recipient's self-identity and capacity for self-determination. According to Seale (1996), older people strive both to maintain a sense of living a meaningful life and to keep their 'reputation' safe, with reputation being based primarily on being perceived as independent in three important areas: self-care, maintaining an orderly physical environment and sustaining social relationships.

Seale (1996) argues that family carers engage in two sets of activities, one to reinforce perceptions of independence and the other to reduce risk. These are 'surveillance' and 'placement'. Surveillance involves keeping an eye on the older person and 'placement' the initiation of additional support, and ultimately possible admission to alternative care, if safety is unacceptably compromised. However, achieving an appropriate balance between these activities is important for if older people feel that their self-identity is threatened or their 'reputation' is compromised then they resist offers of support and may consequently be labelled as 'difficult', particularly by formal service providers. According to Seale (1996), carers occupy an ambiguous position as by providing support they may simultaneously create dependency. The challenge therefore is to provide care in such a way so as to maintain a sense of independence and reciprocation in the caring dynamic. This requires creativity and imagination and, particularly for formal service providers, a willingness to conceptualize roles in more innovative ways.

Conversely, although carers may be in a position of power with respect to care-recipients, this is not always the case. There is growing evidence that formal carers are sensitive to the reactions of older people and that older people are often aware of the need to be sensitive to the reactions of family carers. Cox and Dooley (1996), in one of the few studies to explore simultaneously the views of care-receivers and caregivers, interviewed 91 care-receivers (31 black, 30 Hispanic and 30 white) about their perceptions of their role. They found that most care-receivers found it difficult to accept their need for help due to the high societal value placed upon independence. Consequently many reported feelings of being a burden, feeling guilty about needing help and struggling to maintain independence. There was also recognition of the need for help and a realization that if equitable relationships with family carers were to be maintained then they needed to work collaboratively with those giving care. Care-receivers therefore tried to be as self-caring as possible; not to be too demanding; not to complain too much; to keep their requests to a minimum; to let the carer know their help was appreciated; to give love to the carer; to talk to the carer about their needs. These data accurately reflect many of the satisfactions reported by caregivers themselves (Nolan *et al.* 1996a; Grant *et al.* 1998) and suggest that in many cases care-receivers become skilled in maintaining delicate and subtle reciprocities in relationships.

Interestingly caregivers in the same study (Cox and Dooley 1996) identified a similar set of factors that made caregiving either easier or more difficult. Generally care-receivers whom it was relatively easy to support: tried to help as much as possible; provided emotional support to the caregiver; were appreciative; had a sense of humour; were fun to be with; and did not complain. Conversely it was seen as difficult to provide care to someone who: resisted the need for help from either family or professionals; had no interest; was too demanding; or expected more than the caregiver could provide.

On the basis of their study Cox and Dooley (1996) identified three general styles of interaction between caregivers and care-receivers:

- positive and proactive
- passive and accepting
- angry, negative and demanding.

They argued that more empirical studies are required to elaborate further upon their results but believe they provide growing support of the need to understand the often delicate and reciprocal dynamics that occur between caregivers and care-receivers.

Complementing the above findings, there is also increasing awareness of the importance of relationships between formal care providers and both family caregivers and older care-receivers. The difficulties that family carers experience in their relationships with service agencies have already been considered in Chapter 2 and much of our current thinking has been influenced by the work of Twigg and Atkin (1994). The increased emphasis now being placed on working in partnership with family carers (Askham 1998; Banks 1999; Department of Health 1999a) challenges formal providers to be more explicit in their rationale for working with family carers. Complementing, but not explicitly building on the work of Twigg and Atkin (1994), other studies have also highlighted the need for more informed interactions between formal and family carers.

For example, Brown *et al.* (1996b) from the perspective of occupational therapists identified seven potential levels of interaction with family carers, as follows:

- No involvement — relationships based on a traditional medical model with a focus on the patient only
- Family as informant — a passive role for the family, purely as a source of information
- Family as therapy assistant — traditional role in rehabilitation where the family is seen as a resource useful in facilitating the rehabilitation process
- Family as co-client — where the focus of intervention is on the whole family unit
- Family as consultant — with the family playing a much more active role in goal planning, but not as a full member of the multidisciplinary team
- Family as collaborator — included as a full member of the multidisciplinary team
- family as director — where the family takes the lead role, with the OT acting as a resource and facilitator.

Brown *et al.* (1996b) argue that OTs should be more sensitive to the changing involvement of the family over time and that their training should better equip them with the skills and knowledge necessary to work more productively with family carers.

Similarly Hasselkus (1994), also an occupational therapist, charts the changing involvement of the family in the rehabilitation of older people. She outlines three models based primarily on the stages of rehabilitation.

- In the early stages the professional is largely the 'expert' whose role is to help the family to develop their own knowledge and skills.
- At the time of discharge from hospital the family is seen as an equal partner.
- Upon return home the family take the lead role and assume the role of expert.

Hasselkus (1994) does not see relationships as static and linear, but rather describes them as a 'dance' where the relative contribution shifts over time. She believes that the primary role of occupational therapists is to help carers get ready to 'take over' and argues that therapists should not feel threatened or usurped by this. This is seen to require a reorientation of professional training.

Hasselkus's (1994) conclusions are consistent with the 'carers as experts' approach (Nolan *et al.* 1996a) and also resonate closely with other work from the United States based upon the concept of caregiving preparedness (Archbold *et al.* 1992). More recent work by Schumacher *et al.* (1998) elaborates upon many of these concepts, arguing that the ability of the family to care 'well' is central to the success of community care in the United

States. They highlight the desire of family carers to do a 'good job' but also describe their fears that they may lack the necessary skills and knowledge. Schumacher *et al.* (1998) promote the need for a fuller understanding of what it means to 'do caring well' and explore further a number of related concepts such as mastering self-efficacy, competence, preparedness and ability. On the basis of their review they conclude that the above concepts require further refinement and elaboration in order to inform the role of professional interventions in helping carers to care well.

While the above studies signal the need for a more comprehensive understanding of the interactions between family and formal caregivers, recent work from Sweden (Ingvad and Olsson 1999; Olsson and Ingvad 1999) draws attention to the delicate dynamics that often exist between older people and home carers. These authors describe a diverse and complex range of practical, social and emotional exchanges that occur. Positive and reciprocal relationships are more likely to develop when the home carer feels appreciated and valued by the older person and has their competencies and skills recognized. Conversely if older people are seen as indifferent, negative, nagging, demanding, grumbling or ungrateful, then negative relationships are far more likely. These authors argue that some 'sharing' of personal experiences is important to the development of positive relationships and that trust and confidence based on a congruent set of expectations are essential. This is far more likely when there is continuity of relationships over time. Furthermore, as there is often very little in the way of physical improvement among older people in receipt of home care, Ingvad and Olsson (1999) argue that care-receiver satisfaction with the support they receive is an integral part of job satisfaction for the home carer, highlighting the need for far greater attention to be given to the emotional climate of the exchange (Olsson and Ingvad 1999).

The congruence between these results, those of Cox and Dooley (1996) and the satisfactions of caring described in a number of studies (Nolan *et al.* 1996a; Grant *et al.* 1998) not only indicates an emerging consensus, but also highlights the need for further empirical work in this area. This is particularly important if formal service providers are to be more fully attuned to the delicate reciprocities in family relations and are also to achieve maximum job satisfaction themselves.

Community care and older people: improving service responses

Responding to the diverse needs of an increasing large population of older people and their family carers in the context of current policy initiatives promoting independence raises a number of issues. These relate both to the way that services are organized and delivered and how service providers are trained and educated. A consideration of the role of community nursing, and district nursing in particular, provides an elegant case example.

In the introduction to the most recent National Strategy on Nursing in England (Department of Health 1999c), the then Minister for Health, Frank Dobson, stressed the central role that nursing will play in achieving the policy aspirations of the government. The document outlines the changing context of care delivery, emphasizing the ageing population, the need for better management of chronic illnesses, more efficient strategies for health promotion and the importance of working with family carers. In responding to this ambitious agenda, new roles for nurses in primary and community care are described addressing health equalities and social exclusion, promoting health and supporting carers. While many would endorse such roles, a comprehensive review of the district nursing service undertaken by the Audit Commission (1999) indicates the significant challenges that such initiatives face.

The review begins by presenting statistics suggesting that district nurses provide most of the nursing and related care in the community, visiting 2.75 million people annually, amounting to 36 million patient contacts. The majority of these contacts are with frail older people, with over half the population aged 85 plus being visited by a district nurse. Despite this level of contact the review concludes that district nursing is a comparatively under-researched area. Nevertheless changes in patterns of service delivery are evident. District nurses increasingly work at the boundaries between health and social care, with a year-on-year increase in the numbers of frail older people visited. Due to faster patient through-put from acute care, however, there is a growing emphasis on technical as opposed to personal aspects of nursing. This raises significant questions about who district nurses should support, where their efforts are most appropriately directed, and what knowledge and skills are required to deliver optimum care.

The review gave particular consideration to the importance of a thorough and comprehensive assessment, using leg ulcers and continence as case examples. The audit revealed wide variations in practice with important elements of the assessment process often being deficient. In relation to incontinence, for example, a conservative approach was often in evidence, with a focus on managing the problem rather than proactively identifying and treating the cause. Only half of the assessments reviewed had ruled out infection as a potential factor either aggravating or causing the incontinence, and frequency and volume of urine were considered in only one out of six cases.

Furthermore while deficiencies in the technical components of care were apparent, tensions also emerged in the interpersonal aspects. The review described how the humanity of the district nursing service was seen as fundamentally important by patients and carers, stressing that a one-to-one relationship with an individual who could be respected and trusted was essential to quality of care. However, the growing focus on technical nursing was seen to threaten these crucial, interactional components of care.

> These are not added extras but are essential to a sense of personal security and quality of life for people living with illness, disability and deteriorating health. Trusts and commissioners should recognise that with pressures on services to increase efficiency and the rise in technical as opposed to personal nursing care, there is a danger that some of the things that patients say they value most will be lost.
>
> (Audit Commission 1999: 53–4)

The need to capture these less tangible elements of care in future national surveys of users' experiences was stressed but somewhat paradoxically the review later suggested that many of the 'more routine nursing tasks' could be delegated to nursing assistants. As highlighted in Chapter 3, it is largely in the context of care delivery that interpersonal dynamics are acted out. To argue that such care can be more appropriately delivered by unqualified staff seems to directly contradict the sentiments evident in the above quotation.

In its conclusion the Audit Commission (1999) identified a number of factors affecting the district nursing service which, with minor variations, could apply equally not only to health care more generally but also to social services. These include the increasingly complex packages of care delivered in the community, incorporating both palliative and terminal care and the rise in dependency levels, which have been exacerbated since 1990. In responding to these factors it was seen as essential to maintain the confidence and trust that patients and carers have in the district nursing service and to recognize the value they place on the 'human' aspects of service delivery, that is, on feeling cared for and having someone to listen to concerns and worries. Such aspects were seen currently to be under threat by the expectations that services provide 'more for less' with the consequent tendency to redraw boundaries and focus on specific tasks to the detriment of patient centred care.

Interestingly these tensions closely mirror those identified in Chapter 3, particularly the importance of practitioners demonstrating both technical and interpersonal competence. As with the literature on acute care, there are deficiencies in both these areas, as confirmed by the empirical studies cited earlier in this chapter based on the views of older people, carers and front-line practitioners (Easterbrook 1999; Farell *et al.* 1999). Developing appropriate responses to these tensions provides one of the main challenges to practitioners and policy makers in acute, rehabilitative and community contexts, well into the new millennium.

5

The care needs of older people and family caregivers in continuing care settings

Sue Davies

A sizeable minority of older people are likely to need special care as they grow more frail (Royal Commission on Long-Term Care 1999). Most of these people will continue to be cared for in their own homes, usually with the support of family and friends complemented by statutory services. Meanwhile, the demand for residential and nursing home care continues to rise; there are currently nearly half a million people residing in care homes or long-term hospital care.

Historically, work within such environments has not been given a high status nor seen as requiring much skill. On the contrary, creating a positive environment for continuing care is a highly demanding and skilful job and there is a growing awareness that many long-term care homes in the UK are failing to meet the needs of older people in their care. Campaigns by organizations representing older people and reports in the media have continued to highlight inadequate care in both the private and statutory sectors with the consequence that entry to a care home is commonly viewed as an 'unavoidable spectre facing those in their later years' (Biedenheim and Normoyle 1991: 107). This chapter aims to draw together literature describing the experiences of older people living in care homes, their families and staff working in these environments, in order to present a more balanced view and to identify a framework to guide practice which will help ensure a good quality of life for older people living in care homes.

A note on methods

Exploration of the literature on continuing care for older people identified items from the fields of nursing, medicine, social gerontology, social work and psychology (see Appendix). Synthesis of this diverse literature has focused upon the experiences of residents, family caregivers and staff in order to identify strategies which practitioners can use to enhance the quality of life of residents of care homes, while also supporting family caregivers in the most appropriate way. To complement the review of the literature, semi-structured interviews were conducted with eleven residents in three nursing homes. The intention was to consider the extent to which the themes emerging from the review resonated with the experiences of older people themselves. Additionally, the transcripts of ten interviews with relatives of older people living in nursing homes were examined. These interviews were carried out as part of a study exploring relatives' experiences of nursing home entry and included interviews with four community dwelling spouses, five adult children and one nephew who was the primary family caregiver for his aunt. Finally, the themes were discussed with five practitioners working in the field of continuing care for older people. Quotes from these interviews are incorporated within the chapter to illustrate the key themes.

Focus of this review

Many older people who need regular or continuous care are able to remain in their own homes, often with support from family caregivers complemented by paid carers and health professionals. The implications for health and social care interventions to assist people in these situations is covered in Chapter 4. The main purpose of this chapter is to consider a new approach to the care of older people living in care homes, both residential and nursing. However, the chapter would be incomplete without a brief consideration of some of the alternatives to 'institutional living' and these are discussed within the concluding section. Management of the physical care needs of older people living in care homes, such as the need for continence care, nutrition and skin care, has been ably covered in other texts (see for example Heath and Ford 1996; Bartlett and Burnip 1998). These topics are not covered here in detail; rather the focus is upon the whole experience of moving into and living in a care home and how that experience can be enhanced for older people and their carers.

Policy context

A number of themes can be traced through the policy initiatives of the late twentieth century which have shaped the current experiences of older people living in care homes and their family caregivers. These include an emphasis on widening the choices available to older people in need of continuing care by offering a range of care options, and ensuring that older people receive the right amount of care and support to maintain maximum independence (Reed and Payton 1998). Where older people decide to move into some form of residential care, the emphasis is on creating a homely environment which maximizes opportunities for both social engagement and privacy. However, the extent to which policy initiatives have been successful in achieving these goals is determined largely by financial constraints (Pearson *et al.* 1998). In 1990, the NHS and Community Care Act (Department of Health 1990) introduced a contract culture to arrangements for continuing care, and attempted to promote a mixed economy of care with social services departments purchasing packages of care from a range of service providers. A stated intention of the Act was to increase flexibility and consumer choice. In the absence of any direct purchasing power for consumers, there are concerns that this aim has not been achieved (Impallomeni and Starr 1995; Walker 1999). A report published by an independent firm of financial consultants in 1998 found wide discrepancies between the level of state funding for continuing care and the economic cost of providing such care (Laing 1998). Shortfalls between the level of funding which local authority social services departments will allow for residential and nursing home placements and the fees charged by many care homes have resulted in a two-tier system, where those able to 'top-up' social services payments from their own resources can choose from a wider range of homes.

One of the main consequences of the NHS reforms of the late 1980s and early 1990s has been the widescale relocation of older people from NHS beds to nursing homes in the private sector. The 1980s saw a huge expansion in the number of privately owned nursing homes, many of which went out of business following the 1991 reforms and the tightening up of funding requirements. As a consequence the proportion of homes managed by large corporations is now increasing; this has the advantage of enabling staff to have improved access to support services and programmes of professional development. None the less, the market remains very fluid with 56 per cent of private homes having been open for less than ten years (Bartlett and Burnip 1998).

In view of the concerns which were being expressed over the cost of long-term care and the quality of care in some care homes, the Labour government set up a Royal Commission on Long-Term Care in 1997 under the chairmanship of Sir Stewart Sutherland. The main aim of the commission was to examine the short- and long-term options for a sustainable system of funding of long-term care for elderly people, both in their own homes and in other settings. The commission's main recommendations related to funding arrangements and the key proposal was that nursing care should be centrally funded for all needing long-term care, although means-testing should remain for accommodation and food costs. The commission also made a number of recommendations about the quality of care in nursing homes and proposed the setting up of a National Care Commission with a remit to monitor implementation of the new system, give information and monitor standards. Other recommendations were for nurses to be more involved in assessments for entry to care homes and importantly that services for ethnic minority users should be improved (Royal Commission on Long-Term Care 1999).

To date, the focus of legislation and health authority guidance has been largely on adequacy and quality assurance rather than quality of life (Bartlett and Burnip 1998). Furthermore, there is wide variability in standards and registration requirements between registering health authorities with the consequence that older people residing in different parts of the country are likely to have access to different standards of care (Royal College of Nursing 1994). During 1999, benchmark standards for care and accommodation in nursing and residential homes were developed (Centre for Policy on Ageing 1999). Concerns have been expressed that these standards are unrealistic, particularly in relation to skill mix and room size, and there are fears that homes will be forced to close if the standards become a statutory requirement (Nazarko 1998).

The half-million older people in homes in 2000 are, on average, ten years older than their equivalents in 1990 and significantly more dependent; yet the care home industry relies on nearly one million, mostly untrained staff. It is clear that these staff need effective leadership and high professional standards if the residents of care homes are to maintain a reasonable quality of life. Furthermore, there is an urgent need for a thorough review of the evidence in this field to provide a foundation for education and practice. That is the main purpose of this chapter.

Experiences of life in a care home

A growing body of evidence describes the experience of living in a care home from the older person's perspective and an appreciation of this literature is essential if care is to be truly user-orientated. A range of experiences are described but it is clear that, at its worst, life in a care home is characterized by a sense of powerlessness, vulnerability and loss of meaning (Nystrom and Segesten 1994; Casey and Holmes 1995). Numerous studies and anecdotal accounts over several decades have described how older people are stripped of their identity on admission to a care home (Robb 1967; Laird 1982; Nystrom and Segesten 1990). These experiences are confirmed by the findings of a series of observational studies reporting low levels of staff–resident interaction and minimal involvement in social activities in a range of settings providing continuing care (Armstrong-Esther *et al.* 1994; Gilloran *et al.* 1994; Nolan *et al.* 1995a).

In interviews with 31 residents of two nursing homes in Finland, Liukkonen (1995) found that nursing staff were clearly preoccupied with daily activities, whereas the lives of elderly residents received less attention. There was a widespread feeling among residents that staff members were always pressed for time and did not want to talk with them. However, what these residents wanted most was someone in their daily lives who would 'share with them their joys and sorrows and reminisce with them'. A study of 428 residents of four different care environments, including nursing homes, found high ratings for items relating to medical/technical competence of caregivers and physical-technical conditions of the care environment, but much lower ratings for interpersonal dimensions of care (Wilde *et al.* 1995). A smaller qualitative study of 46 residents of one US nursing home found that the quality of interpersonal relationships with staff members was the most important aspect of quality of care for the residents (Grau *et al.* 1995). In combination, the findings of these studies suggest that while most older people living in care homes feel that their needs for physical care are largely met, care aimed at maintaining their psychological well-being is more elusive.

Islands of the old

Many of the experiences of nursing home life can be seen as the direct consequence of the isolation of nursing homes from the communities in which they are situated. Indeed there are suggestions that older people experience social exclusion following admission to a care home (Royal Commission on Long-Term Care 1999). Adapting Sontag's notion of 'the island of the ill' – a metaphorical and attitudinal place in which we put the sick – Reed (1998) suggests that we have created islands of the old within our society.

> They can wave to us from their shores and we might wave back if we have time, but being ill is being in a different place, and once you've made that journey, it's difficult to get back. Being old seems in many ways similar – we have an island for older people and we like them to go there and stay there.
>
> (Reed 1998: 1)

Islands of the old seems a particularly appropriate metaphor for care homes: many residents have little contact with the outside world and links with local communities are often limited. Most residents perceive that they no longer make any valuable contribution to society. Furthermore, there is evidence of a gap in understanding between the older residents of care homes and the staff caring for them in terms of perceptions of need. A recurrent theme within the literature is that caregivers hold different priorities for frail older people in their care than older people have for themselves (Bartlett 1993; Bliesmer and Earle 1993; Bowsher 1994; Oleson *et al.* 1994).

Staff in care homes also experience isolation and exclusion: terms and conditions of employment are usually inferior to similar work in the statutory sector, opportunities to meet with colleagues in other homes are rare and many staff lack basic preparation for their role. However, the image of care homes as islands of the old can be adapted to more positive effect if we use it to construct ways of improving the lived experience of older people living in care homes. Reed (1998) for example argues that an important aim of nursing home care should be to 'build bridges' between care homes and the wider communities within which they are situated. On the basis of the literature reviewed for this chapter, it is possible to discern a number of themes for improving the experience of older people living in care homes which fit well with the idea of building bridges. These are:

- managing the transition to a care home
- creating a sense of community within a care home
- working to reduce residents' sense of vulnerability and powerlessness
- working to help residents maintain their identity
- maintaining links to family and community.

Each of these objectives will now be considered with reference to the relevant literature and illustrated, where appropriate, with quotes from the interviews with older residents, family members and practitioners.

Managing the transition to a care home

There is no doubt that older people experience profound psychological and physical effects on moving into a care home, but there is evidence that the move can be perceived positively if planned carefully with the involvement of the older person and their family (Nolan *et al.* 1996b; Pearson *et al.* 1998). Studies of the transition to life in a care home have identified the need for continuity of care planning between care settings and there are suggestions that better comprehension of what happens to older patients across organizational boundaries may facilitate continuity of care for older people (Cotter *et al.* 1998). Nolan *et al.* (1996b) describe a typology of admission to represent the range of experience when older people are admitted to a care home. These vary from the positive choice (seen as the ideal) through the rationalized alternative and the discredited option to the fait accompli. Nolan *et al.* suggest that the type of admission experienced by an older person and their family caregivers is influenced by four sets of processes (Table 5.1)

In support of this framework, a number of authors have demonstrated the importance of planned admission involving the older person and their family caregivers as far as possible (Nay 1995; Iwasiw *et al.* 1996; Wilson 1997). Iwasiw *et al.* (1996) interviewed twelve new residents of five nursing homes and concluded that those who had felt actively involved in the decision to be admitted found their adjustment to care was easier. The typology described by Nolan *et al.* (1996b) also resonated with the experiences of the older people and relatives who we interviewed. One relative for example described how he felt his aunt had left the decision to move into a care home too late to be able to adjust easily:

Table 5.1 Processes influencing admission to a care home

Anticipation	the extent to which the admission is planned in a proactive way, with discussion occurring well before decisions are needed
Participation	the extent to which both the older person and their carer(s) are involved in the decision-making process
Exploration	in three main areas: • alternatives to admission to care • of feelings towards admission • of a number of possible homes
Information	the extent to which older people and their carers received sufficient information on which to base an informed choice

Source: Nolan *et al.* 1996b

> If she'd gone into a nursing home when she was still a bit more active and not in a crisis situation she would have taken to it more easily, so I think we were right really in trying to encourage her a year or two earlier. But of course by the time she actually got in to the nursing home things had begun to shut down. She'd become too frail, she moved in when she was ill, the deafness had become more of a problem.
>
> *(Nephew)*

Helping older people and their families to make the right choice about care options is an important role for care staff in a wide range of settings. Several of the older residents we interviewed had not been involved in the decision about a home and some had not even had the opportunity to visit the home before they were admitted. On the basis of longitudinal interviews with 46 older people before and after the transition to a nursing home, Reed *et al.* (1998) highlight the importance of 'place' for each individual seeking admission to a care home. In other words, the location of the home should allow residents to share memories of their community with other residents and maintain links with family and friends. Reed and Payton (1998) argue that care staff also need to recognize the hard work that older people perform when they move into a care home in relation to fitting in with existing conventions and rules, what they term 'constructing familiarity and managing the self'.

Older people adapt to life in a nursing home in a variety of ways and support needs to be tailored accordingly (Savishinsky 1991; Reed and Payton 1998). On the basis of staged interviews with six residents during the first year following admission to a nursing home, Patterson (1995) identifies emotional support as a key factor in adjustment. In one of the few papers to apply a specific theoretical model to the needs of older people, Oleson and Shadick (1993) consider the relevance of Moos and Schaefer's (1986) model of life crises and transitions in supporting adjustment. On the basis of the model Oleson and Shadick (1993) suggest that staff in care homes should

- establish the meaning and understand the personal significance of the situation to the resident
- help the resident to confront reality and respond to the requirements of the situation
- assist the resident to sustain relationships with family members and friends as well as other individuals who may be helpful in resolving the crisis and its aftermath
- help to maintain a reasonable emotional balance by managing upsetting feelings aroused by the situation
- preserve a satisfactory self-image and maintain a sense of competence and mastery.

Adjustment is likely to be made easier if the exact purpose and nature of the admission has been clearly discussed and agreed with the older person and their family. Increasingly, admission to a care home may not necessarily be a permanent decision and the role of nursing homes in providing respite care and rehabilitation is gradually expanding (Baltes *et al.* 1994; Salgado *et al.* 1995; Blair *et al.* 1996).

Creating a sense of community within a care home

Quality of life in a care home setting has been described as 'a lived experience that has both personal and community dimensions' (Brown and Thompson 1994: 132). Certainly, the prospect of social exclusion following admission to a care home can be diminished if this represents simply a move from one community to another, particularly if the care home also has a role within a wider community. However, if we are to create true communities within nursing homes, the complexity and reciprocity within family caregiving relationships needs to be mirrored within the care home environment (Savishinsky 1991). There is firm evidence to suggest that perceptions of quality of care among residents are closely linked to the nature of interpersonal relationships with staff (Powers 1992; Grau *et al.* 1995; Haap *et al.* 1996). For example, in interviews with 46 nursing home residents, Grau *et al.* (1995) found that the vast majority of both positive and negative experiences recalled by residents were concerned primarily with the quality of interpersonal relationships and the sensitivity and kindness (or their opposites) of care personnel. Studies have also highlighted the importance of interactions with staff in reducing agitation among nursing home residents (Cohen-Mansfield *et al.* 1992; Ragneskog *et al.* 1998).

Nolan and Grant (1993) highlight the importance of reciprocity within caregiving relationships for staff, particularly in reducing occupational burnout. However, systems for organizing caregiving, such as named nursing and key worker systems, which could encourage and support relationships between staff and residents are often resisted. For example, an audit of care plans for 298 residents in 17 care homes in the UK found that fewer than half of the residents had a key worker (Brocklehurst and Dickinson 1996). This is in spite of evidence to suggest that consistent staff allocation results in greater resident satisfaction with care (Patchner and Patchner 1993; Teresi *et al.* 1993).

Residents also need opportunities to build relationships with other residents and their families (Powers 1991; Patterson 1995; Reed and Payton 1998). Kovach for example interviewed 50 elderly residents of six nursing homes (Kovach and Robinson 1996) and found a relationship between room-mate rapport and life satisfaction for those who were able to converse. Doyle (1995) also found a significant relationship between absence of close friends among other residents and depressive symptoms. Yet staff in care homes frequently fail to recognize the significance of the relationships which residents have with each other (Reed 1998). This was confirmed in our interviews:

> Well there's a table next to us and there's two women – and they're terrible. They sit staring at us. Well they've put one of them on our table this morning and we weren't very pleased with that. Our names are meant to be on our table. There's five of us on our table and we're all comfortable. But she spoilt it this morning.

The importance of meal-times and dining together as a social event has been demonstrated in the literature (Liukkonen 1995; Kayser Jones 1996). For residents with severe functional impairment, dining with other residents who are able to eat independently has been shown to improve self-feeding (Van Ort and Phillips 1995). Soothing dinner music has also been shown to alter residents' behaviour at meal-times (Ragneskog *et al.* 1996; Denney 1997). For example, Ragneskog *et al.* (1996) found that music at meal-times calmed residents who were agitated and encouraged increased nutritional intake. Residents also spent longer at meals.

Opportunities for shared activities help to create a sense of community and can improve quality of life and cognitive functioning (Turner 1993). Hall and Bocksnick (1995) caution against compelling residents to take part, however; Laird (1982) provides a vivid account of the consequences of inappropriate group activities for residents. Our interviews suggested that in some homes, activities were available only to a select minority and that this was largely due to staff shortages. There is very little in the literature concerning the role of designated activity coordinators within care homes, although a survey of 200 Australian nursing homes found a positive relationship between the presence of an activities coordinator and the range of experiences enjoyed by residents (Pearson *et al.* 1992).

Another frequently ignored factor in developing a sense of community within a care home relates to helping residents and staff to come to terms with death and bereavement (Nolan and Keady 1996). The unavoidable confrontation with the processes of death and dying associated with life in a nursing home have been linked with high levels of depression among residents (Abrams *et al.* 1992). High mortality rates in nursing homes are also stressful for staff: 'I think that's unique, for any person to deal with 60 deaths a year – of people they have become close to' (Nursing home manager).

Commemorating death and carrying out rituals which remind and demonstrate to others that a death has occurred is an important way of sensitizing people to loss and also challenges the denial of death (Costello 1996). However, the literature revealed few studies which have considered the support needed by residents and staff following the death of a resident. One North American study (Murphy *et al.* 1997) considered the bereavement services available for families of older people with Alzheimer's disease living in long-term care facilities. A survey of 121 nursing homes revealed that 98 per cent of homes did not visit, make phone calls or provide written information to family members in the period following a resident's death. This is obviously an area needing further research.

Finally, building a community within a care home is dependent upon creating a sense of 'home' for residents, a feeling that they belong and have rights and responsibilities. This was vividly captured by a nursing home manager in one of our interviews, who described how a resident had greeted the manager's husband when he visited the home:

> They were in this little tea-bar and I took my husband round and I introduced him to this lady and she offered him a cup of tea and I thought that was brilliant because that's how it should be because it's her home not mine, and she saw it as her place to offer hospitality.
>
> (Nursing home manager)

Working to reduce residents' sense of vulnerability and powerlessness

The vulnerability which older people feel as a result of their dependence on nursing home staff has been vividly described in many first-hand accounts (Laird 1982; Nystrom and Segesten 1994; Reed and Payton 1998) and was also reflected within our interviews:

> You've got to have a bath whether you like it or not. They tell you in the morning whether you are having a bath or not.

> I don't use the commode very often at night – on average about twice. To me, I'm a little bit on the nervous side and there's one – she's always rushing me. The other night I said, 'Oh for goodness sake go out a bit',

because if they go out I can manage. Now some of them are very, very good – they say, 'Oh we'll just have a little walk' and it's all the difference. But this one – she burst out the other night, went straight to the sister and complained about me and the sister came in here and she thoroughly tore me a strip off which I thought wasn't very nice. I mean I pay my money to be looked after, not to be dictated to.

Care staff are in a position to act as gatekeepers to essential care (Herzberg 1993), medical care (Gillick and Mendes 1996), pain control (Ferrell 1995) and opportunities for social interaction (Gilloran *et al.* 1994; Nolan *et al.* 1995a). The regular exclusion of older people and their families from discussions about their care and progress is a further example of the ways in which older people living in nursing homes are disempowered. Yet involvement in decision making has positive benefits for the residents of nursing homes, with several studies demonstrating a relationship between the maintenance of personal control and resident outcomes such as psychological well-being and satisfaction with care (Bowsher and Gerlach 1990; Beery 1993; Chen and Snyder 1996; Warner 1997). Chen and Snyder (1996) for example found that residents' perception of personal control explained 54 per cent of the variance in satisfaction with care. Providing opportunities for residents to make even small choices and decisions regarding their daily lives can increase their perception of autonomy and control, both of which are often severely curtailed in an institutional environment (Goodwinjohansson 1996). Perceptions of the potential loss of personal autonomy may also influence decision making about care options: in a survey of preferences for continuing care, loss of control was cited as the main reason participants would not choose entry to a care home as a preferred care option (Kelly *et al.* 1998).

The sense of vulnerability felt by many frail older people living in care homes can be compounded by communication problems. Numerous studies for example have found high levels of hearing loss among residents of nursing homes (Mahoney 1992; Stumer *et al.* 1996; Tolson and McIntosh 1997). On the basis of a review of the mainly US literature in this field, Lubinski (1995) suggests there is likely to be little communicative interaction in nursing homes and that communication, when it does occur is likely to be impoverished. This is attributed to a range of factors including:

- the paucity of communication services to meet the needs of residents
- barriers to the uptake of services including cognitive impairment of residents
- physical health problems and the lack of access to on-site hearing tests coupled with the expense of travel to off-site assessment and treatment.

The potential resource implications for overcoming these barriers suggest that initiatives within the home are likely to be more successful in improving residents' ability to communicate and a number of evaluation studies have demonstrated improvements in communication following structured intervention programmes (Buckwalter *et al.* 1991; Jordan *et al.* 1993). Jordan *et al.* (1993) found positive gains in communication skills and self-management of communicative impairment for a number of residents following intervention programmes implemented by volunteers. Similarly, Buckwalter *et al.* (1989) found that dedicated, ten-minute communication interventions by nurses increased the ability of older residents to interact. Modifying the 'listening environment' through strategies such as rescheduling cleaning activities have also been shown to be effective in improving communicative ability (Tolson and McIntosh 1997). Finally, there may also be a role for independent advocates in improving communication between professionals and older residents (Evans 1994).

An older person's right to self-determination is automatically threatened by virtue of living in a care home since the need for care necessarily impinges on autonomy. Nolan *et al.* in Chapter 1 of this book go so far as to suggest that personal autonomy is not always an appropriate goal within the context of a care home where all residents will, to some extent be dependent on care staff (see Chapter 1, this volume). After Clark (1995), they contend that the values of community, collectiveness and interdependence are more relevant guides for practice. A nursing home manager we interviewed also questioned the way in which the concept of independence is operationalized within the context of nursing home care:

> When people talk about independence in nursing homes, you know they're saying you're independent if you can wash your face, whereas really it's much deeper than that. You're independent if you can say to the nurse, 'Please come here and wash my face'.
>
> (Nursing home manager)

If older people living in care homes are to retain a sense of control over their lives, there is a need to reconceptualize caring so that staff become supporters and advocates for older people rather than custodians and guardians. Residents must be encouraged to become active partners rather than passive recipients of care. There is also a need to balance risk taking in relation to personal autonomy to ensure that older people feel safe, since many residents identify a sense of safety as one of the main benefits of living in a care home (Raynes 1998).

Working to help residents maintain their identity

Identity is linked closely with the notion of self-esteem, which has been described as one of the main ingredients of quality of life in old age:

> Positive self-esteem is a sense of integrity and identity, founded on connections to the person one has been, memories, roles, unique qualities, relations, belongings and home.
>
> (Nystrom and Segesten 1990: 57)

Perhaps more than in any other care environment, it is essential to locate the care of older people living in nursing homes in the context of their whole life development. The importance of building plans of care based on an older person's biography should hardly need to be stated. However, biographical detail within nursing assessment and documentation is often limited (Brocklehurst and Dickinson 1996). There is also evidence that family caregivers are frequently not involved in the care-planning process (Norburn *et al.* 1995). Ford and McCormack (1999) argue that expert nurses are those who appreciate the influences of individual characteristics on care, characteristics such as family relationships, occupation, cultural background, spiritual beliefs and sexuality. However, in the absence of detailed assessment in negotiation with the resident and their family, it is difficult to imagine how these characteristics can influence caregiving.

The significance to residents of staff recognizing their individuality was apparent in our interviews: 'I don't feel as if I'm just another one – I feel as if I'm still me. They're not just treating me as anybody.'

Another resident described the significance of carers recognizing things that were important to her:

> The other week, there's someone here – her cat had kittens and one of the helpers – she was having one of these kittens and I had to have mine rehomed when I moved in here and I'm very fond of animals. They were handing it over here so I said 'I want to see it'. And they brought that kitten in to see me and I nursed it. It made my day.

Cookman (1996) describes how things, places, animals and ideas can be sources of security, belonging and self-identity for older people and argues that care staff need to see the environment of the care home as a supportive resource, for example using objects to induce reminiscence. Objects can also be used to remind staff of the older person's background and interests. One spouse described how the manager of her husband's nursing home had asked her to bring in some of the items of furniture he had made before he was disabled by Parkinson's disease.

> He said 'I wonder if you could bring a few of the things down that he's made', because they were having a meeting with some of the carers and nurses about Parkinson's. And he thought this would show how Peter was before he was ill. Because they just know him as sitting there, kind of thing. So when J came that weekend we took quite a few things down that he'd made . . . because then everybody realizes how talented he is.
>
> (Wife of resident)

The significance to families of working to maintain a resident's identity was also apparent in our interviews with relatives:

> When she's lost her glasses, and this has happened about a dozen times since I've been there, and at the moment her glasses have gone.

Yesterday when I went, she hadn't even got her own glasses on, she'd got somebody else's. And I understand that there are patients and nurses that if they see anything then they'll pick it up, but I do feel that they could be more diligent in that respect. Things like I went in the other week and I found a woman with Daisy's clothes on. And that upset me.

(Husband of resident)

In terms of helping an older person to maintain their identity, the importance of 'knowing the person' is clear (Evans 1996; McCormack and Ford 1999b). Consistent staff assignment is one way of ensuring that staff are familiar with a resident's personal history and preferences. Osberg *et al.* (1987) also highlight the importance of intimacy in helping residents to maintain a sense of their own identity. They argue that, while it is often impossible to improve functional and cognitive ability for highly dependent residents of nursing homes, it should be possible to increase the quantity and depth of social and non-sexual physical intimacy. They suggest that this is likely to result in improvements in quality of life.

The importance of recognizing cultural factors in helping residents of care homes to maintain a sense of identity has received scant attention in the literature. One example of an educational programme to develop culturally appropriate care in nursing homes is described by Reynolds (1992), who suggests five domains where practitioners need to be particularly aware of cultural preferences. These are communication and language, personal space (proximity and comfort), time (flexibility in relation to routine), social organization (recognizing family ties and how best to support family members) and environmental control (for example retaining opportunities to engage in culturally specific practices such as folk medicine).

The role of meaningful activity in helping residents to retain their sense of identity is also apparent within the literature (Laird 1982; Daley 1993). Furthermore, a key theme to emerge from the interviews with residents was a wish for more activities. Those residents who were taken on outings enjoyed themselves and wished that these could happen more often: 'They took me out in the bus into Derbyshire and do you know, I never thought I would see it again. It was wonderful'.

Time to chat with staff is highly valued but appears to happen less frequently than residents would like.

I don't get no company: that's the point I'm on my own. I might as well be at home in my own bedroom. People don't take the time to talk. That's the trouble, I've nobody to talk to. I'm on my own so much and I like a bit of company. I've nobody at home. Nobody comes now to see me. Still I suppose they have other things to do.

Even when staff do not have the resources for formal activities and outings, just 'popping in' to check that residents are all right is appreciated.

I'd like someone to occasionally come in to see if there's anything I want doing. Even if it's only a few minutes, say ten minutes or so just to sort things out a little bit. It doesn't need to be at a fixed time – any-time would be all right – I'm always at home.

This contrasted with the experience of another resident, who found that staff made time to call in to 'chat' with her:

They don't just come in and do a job and go out – they're speaking, have a little chat. I mean this lunch-time they came to collect my tray and she said, 'Oh you're doing the crossword.' So I passed it over and said, 'Here you are – have a go.' And it's just the minute or two they spare and it means a lot.

Nystrom and Segesten (1990) provide an additional dimension to aid an understanding of what constitutes quality of life in frail old age. On the basis of qualitative interviews with residents, they describe three hierarchical levels in relation to what healthy living means to older people residing in nursing homes:

1 Daily life worthy of human beings – acceptable daily functioning, a pleasant environment and relief from pain and worries.
2 Positive self-esteem – identity and integrity.
3 An experience of peace of mind.

In particular the authors identify peace of mind as a key element of health which, if present, is able to transcend shortcomings in other areas. In a follow-up study (Nystrom and Segesten 1995), thirteen registered nurses employed in five nursing homes within one Swedish city were asked how they could support the attainment of this state of mind in elderly, lucid patients. Four different aspects of nursing support through interaction were identified:

• support through instrumental activities (respect, dignity, independence)
• support through daily coexistence (normalizing, creating a homely environment)
• support through genuine encounters (reaching, coming close to, developing a trusting relationship, encountering the resident as a human being)
• support through empowering supportive interventions (understanding a person's background and taking risks).

While this is a small study based upon the perspective of nurses, these functions are worthy of further research.

Maintaining links to family and community

The importance of maintaining family relationships following the move to a nursing home, both for the older person and their family members, has been clearly demonstrated (Bogo 1987; Daley 1993; Gladstone 1995; Ross *et al.* 1997)

In an original study, essays were gathered from 53 elderly nursing home residents about the strongest meaning in their lives (DePaola and Ebersole 1995). Residents most often reported the category of family relationships as central, followed by pleasure and then health. Several studies have considered the role of relatives in nursing homes and have highlighted the need for nursing home staff to be made more aware of relatives' needs (Relatives Association 1997; Morrow-Howell 1998), both at the time of admission and subsequently. Family members experience loss, guilt and grief, following the admission of their relative and report that these emotions continue throughout the time that their older member is in the nursing home (Johnson 1990; Tilse 1994; Dellasega and Mastrian 1995). Contrary to popular perceptions, most relatives wish for continued involvement following admission (Bogo 1987) and there is some evidence that family members want their involvement to be negotiated (Davies *et al.* 1999). However, our interviews with relatives suggested that this is a rare occurrence.

> A few days ago when I went up she had been unwell, but nobody had phoned me to let me know. There's nothing I could have done for her anyway. It would be nice though if they did ring me to let me know, then I could ask if I should be there . . . that would be nice. They also don't make a point of telling me how she has been, I always have to ask.
>
> (Daughter)

Furthermore, care staff frequently fail to recognize and draw upon the expertise of family caregivers in planning and implementing care for the older person (Naleppa 1996), in spite of evidence demonstrating the benefits of involving family members for all concerned (Buckwalter *et al.* 1991; Relatives' Association 1997). In encouraging relative involvement, it is important to recognize the different roles which family caregivers may wish to occupy. On the basis of semi-structured interviews with mainly female adult children, Bowers (1987) identifies five distinct but overlapping categories of family caregiving – anticipatory, supervisory, preventive, instrumental and protective. Staff also need to consider ways to support relatives during visits, particularly where the resident is cognitively impaired and conversation is difficult.

In order to provide the most appropriate care for relatives, staff in care homes must understand family experiences at this time, in particular their need to share feelings with others. The literature reveals a small number of studies which have evaluated more structured approaches to supporting and involving relatives, such as relative support groups, with beneficial outcomes (Drysdale *et al.* 1993; Campbell and Linc 1996; Morrow-Howell 1998). On the basis of a review of the literature in this area, Nolan and Dellasega (1999) identify four potentially useful interventions which might enable residents to maintain relationships with close family and friends in a way that is mutually beneficial:

- Creating a welcoming environment which encourages and supports visiting, and working with carers to maximize their involvement and facilitate a sense of purpose.
- Recognizing and clarifying roles and responsibilities for both groups.
- Valuing and accessing the carer's knowledge and expertise and utilizing this as an important component of planning care.
- Helping carers to create a positive perception of the admission, acknowledging their need to both receive and provide help, and dealing with emotional reactions.

(Nolan and Dellasega 1999)

In relation to the wider community, a number of approaches to bringing community members into the nursing home have been described, although most of the reported schemes are North American. Savishinsky (1991) used an ethnographic approach over several years to explore the effects for residents and staff of a pet therapy programme whereby local people and college students brought companion animals into nursing homes on a weekly basis. Visiting people and pets re-created an 'aura of domesticity for residents' who had been cut off from their homes and families. Concomitantly, most volunteers came to see themselves as family and friends to residents rather than as visitors, strangers or adjunct staff.

Improving the care experience: managing change in care homes

One of the biggest challenges facing practitioners caring for older people in any care setting is the need to change entrenched care practices, which are often based on inappropriate attitudes and beliefs (Mattiasson and Andersson 1994; Gibbs 1995; Jacelon 1995). Several decades of research has continued to demonstrate that 'routine' rather than individualized care is the norm in many settings providing continuing care for older people. Several authors argue that the way to improve care for older people in a range of care environments is to create a culture of positive care which values older people and the staff working with them (Davies *et al.* 1999; McCormack and Wright 1999). Some practical approaches to changing the culture of care are now considered.

Involving users and accessing user views

A growing body of research suggests that there is enormous value in identifying the older person's perspective on caregiving and the need for care and that this should be a basic principle of service provision. In particular, studies suggest that there is often a disparity between nurses' perceptions and the perceptions of older people themselves in relation to priorities for caregiving. This suggests that accessing user views and feeding these views into a change process should be a priority. To date, the involvement of service users and carers in planning, managing and delivering care services and improving the quality of care they receive in the community has not been a central tenet of the delivery of either health or social care in the UK (Raynes 1998). Some recent work has attempted to access user views and feed these directly into the commissioning process (see for example Barnes and Walker 1996; Mitchell and Koch 1997; Raynes 1998; Reed *et al.* 1999). These initiatives demonstrate the importance of allowing adequate time to gain residents' confidence and the need for careful attention to practical details (such as transport arrangements and refreshments) so that the event is a positive experience for those involved. However, they also demonstrate the benefits for service providers and participants of such a collaborative approach. Some of the key points to emerge from such work are shown in Table 5.2.

A small number of studies describe approaches to involving residents and family caregivers more closely in care processes. For example, Ruland *et al.* (1997) describe the use of an assessment tool to measure self-care abilities which records the patient's priorities and any disagreement between them and the assessor about their ability to perform the activities.

Effects of different staffing levels and skill mix on quality of care

A common suggestion for improving the quality of care in nursing homes is to increase the ratio of qualified nurses and reduce the reliance on unqualified health care assistants. However, the literature review revealed a dearth of studies which consider the issue of skill mix within the context of nursing homes. Certainly, few studies have addressed the central issue of whether resident outcomes are affected by the skill mix of the nursing team

Table 5.2 What residents of care care homes want

- Activities in the home
- Provision of opportunities to get out of the home
- Provision of good food, choice in relation to it and the opportunity to make a drink
- Provision of kind and knowledgeable staff
- Access to one's bedroom
- Pleasant company and friendship of other residents
- Continuity of staffing
- Physical comfort of the home
- The availability of support services
- Personal safety in the home
- The availability of aids and adaptations to promote self-care

---

Source: After Raynes 1998

or whether similar outcomes can be achieved by varying skill mix combi-
nations. In a carefully designed study, Pearson *et al.* (1992) surveyed 200
non-government homes in four Australian states and found no relationship
between the proportion of qualified nursing staff and quality of care or quality of life for residents. There was a significant positive relationship between
access to therapy staff and the variety of experience of residents. Exposure
to in-service training for staff, and the leadership style of the most senior
nurse within each facility were also found to influence quality of care.

There is some evidence to suggest that the attitude of carers may be a
more significant factor than staffing levels in determining resident experiences (Booth 1985; Reed 1998). Certainly, increasing the proportion of
qualified nursing staff alone appears to have little impact on quality of
care. Sixsmith *et al.* (1993) studied staff activity in six nursing homes for
elderly mentally ill people, three of which had received additional
resources as part of an initiative aimed at promoting 'positive care'. The
researchers found that the extra resources available within the experimental homes were used largely for routine care, such as resident hygiene,
rather than 'positive', life-enhancing care such as social interaction and
group activities. They conclude that, in order to increase 'positive care', it
is necessary to employ staff with that specific function.

Zinn (1993) found no consistent relationship between staffing levels
and selected quality indicators including prevalence of catheterization,
restraint usage and incidence of pressure sores. Data were drawn from ten
metropolitan areas in the United States and also revealed wide variation
in staff to resident ratios. A large retrospective survey of more than 12,000
nursing home residents in one US state (Bliesmer *et al.* 1998) did find a
relationship between licensed nursing hours (that is, the amount of nursing time provided by qualified nurses) and resident outcomes, including
functional ability, probability of being discharged home and death. However, the sample included acutely ill residents; when limited to chronic
residents, this relationship virtually disappeared.

In one of the few qualitative studies to consider issues related to staffing
within nursing homes, Grau *et al.* (1995) explored residents' perceptions
of their quality of care by asking 46 residents to describe both their best
and worst experiences since nursing home placement. Of particular
relevance to the current discussion is the finding that the most frequently
reported worst experiences concerned care provided by unqualified
nursing aides. However, an important limitation of this study is the
researchers' failure to acknowledge that residents will have had more
experience of care provided by nursing aides and are therefore more likely
to recall critical incidents related to them.

Effectiveness of training

There is a growing body of evidence to suggest that care assistants, through
participation in systematic training programmes, have the potential to

affect positively the quality of care in nursing homes (see for example Taival and Raatikainen 1993; Smith *et al.* 1994). A number of studies have identified the importance of regular training within a structured programme, rather than 'one-off' sessions (Nolan and Keady 1996; Davies and Nolan 1998). There is also firm evidence to suggest that training is most effective if combined with follow up supervision 'on the job' (Stevens *et al.* 1998). A series of small-scale studies have shown that regular clinical supervision increases creativity and personal accomplishment, decreases tedium and burnout, allows a more positive assessment of patients' potential for rehabilitation, improves cooperation with colleagues and increases self-confidence (Brocklehurst 1997). There are also suggestions that clinical supervision may contribute to a reduction in absenteeism.

In terms of identifying their own personal challenges and training needs, nurses working in care homes tend to prioritize clinical nursing issues such as pressure sore risk and medication management and indirect nursing issues such as recruitment and retention of staff, rather than issues relating to quality of life (Morrell *et al.* 1995). Lack of preparation for a managerial role has also been highlighted (Bartlett and Burnip 1998).

Teaching nursing homes

With the closure of continuing care wards in NHS hospitals, many educational centres are developing links with private and voluntary nursing homes in order to offer student placements within this environment. Indeed there is some evidence to suggest that students may be exposed to more positive attitudes and appropriate practices within nursing homes than within long-stay hospital wards (Bowling and Formby 1991). Evaluation of students' experiences within teaching nursing homes in North America indicate that the slower-pace and less-threatening atmosphere of the nursing home facilitate effective teaching (Neil *et al.* 1982; Mezey *et al.* 1988). Together, these factors suggest potentially beneficial outcomes for residents, staff and students of further developing links between educational centres and nursing homes within the private sector. The development of teaching-nursing homes would require the input of sufficient resources to allow the establishment of link roles and adequate preparation of staff.

Caution is also necessary to ensure that meeting the needs of students does not conflict with the prime aim of ensuring a good quality of life for residents (Chilvers and Jones 1997).

Specialist practitioners

Further research is needed to evaluate the contribution of specialist practitioner roles to improving the quality of life for older people in care homes. Several authors have described outreach services with teams of specialists providing advice and support to care home staff (Drysdale *et al.*

1993; Patterson 1995; Bott 1998). Proctor *et al.* (1998) evaluated a teaching intervention by a multidisciplinary outreach team aimed at improving the quality of interaction between staff and residents. The intervention included a seminar programme and the introduction of a behavioural approach to care planning. The researchers found a significant increase in the proportion of time spent in positive interactions between staff and residents, both in terms of direct care and social contact at the end of the intervention. Levels of resident activity also increased. Similarly, Smith *et al.* (1995) report an evaluation of a 'train the trainer' model for developing nurse consultants in the management of mental health problems. A CNS (clinical nurse specialist) trained nurses from long-term care facilities in three separate two-day intensive training sessions. These nurses then used the information and programme materials provided to train additional staff in their own facilities, with the CNS continuing to provide consultation. Of those trained by the programme, 83 per cent reported that they were consulted by their staff regarding a patient's care either during or after the training sessions. While this is encouraging, an important limitation of this study is that the impact of the training model on resident outcomes was not considered.

Alternatives to the nursing home

Given the range of threats to personal identity which are posed by the care home environment, this chapter would be incomplete without a brief consideration of the alternatives to nursing and residential home care. Kane *et al.* (1991) for example report an evaluation of an adult foster scheme in the United States which suggests that foster care compares favourably with nursing home care in relation to quality of life and cost. Adult foster care homes are private residences where a live-in manager cares for between one and five disabled residents. Meals are served with residents and staff eating together and routines are kept to a minimum. The resident manager provides personal care and housekeeping and if necessary other services, such as skilled nursing, can be bought in from home health agencies. In a large study comparing the experiences of foster home residents with residents of nursing homes, foster care residents reported more social activity, even when controlled for disability (Kane *et al.* 1991). Factors considered important included a homelike atmosphere, having a safe supervised place to live, personal assistance, privacy, access to medical care and flexible routines. This type of long-term care provision seems to offer a mainstream alternative to nursing homes. However, an extensive review of the literature failed to reveal any similar initiatives in the UK.

Retirement communities for independent older people, popular in the United States, offer access to 24-hour emergency assistance and companionship through planned activities (Arrington 1997). A number of these facilities have added assisted living facilities allowing older residents to 'age in place'. There are similarities with the system of 'service houses' in the Scandinavian countries which provide care for disabled people with care needs from moderate to severe (Trydegard 1998). Older people can move in to the service house while still relatively independent and can negotiate an increase in the level of service as their need for care increases. However, what is lacking within the literature is any comparison of the different models of service delivery for older people with a particular level of need. In the absence of comparative research, the future direction for continuing care provision is unclear.

Theoretical and methodological critique

Most of the research reviewed is cross-sectional with few longitudinal studies tracing the experiences of older people over time. There is also evidence of sampling bias in a number of studies, the majority using purposive or accidental sampling. Overall, the body of research evidence examined revealed a limited focus on the perceptions of older people themselves, particularly those with any degree of cognitive impairment. The views of minority groups such as gay and lesbian older people and older people from ethnic minorities are notable by their absence. Research carried out in the UK, particularly in nursing homes is limited, with most work originating from the United States and Canada, the Scandinavian countries and Australia.

In terms of the development of theory in relation to the needs of older people living in care homes and their families, a number of conceptual and theoretical frameworks are identified in the literature. However, these are mostly derived from research carried out in settings other than care homes and there is a need for more explicit empirical testing of a range of theoretical ideas within this setting.

In spite of these limitations, the literature reveals a remarkable consensus about the factors which contribute to enabling older people to maintain their quality of life after moving into a care home. These factors will now be summarized.

Conclusion

The literature demonstrates the complexity of ensuring that older people residing in nursing homes enjoy a good quality of life. A consistent theme is the need to ensure that nursing care is tailored to individual needs if older people are to achieve optimal quality of life (Davies *et al*. 1997). This requires comprehensive and regular assessment of needs in collaboration with the older person and their family. The significance of interpersonal relationships, both within and outside the home, also seems clear.

Enabling continuity of resident/staff relationships through the retention of a stable workforce is likely to enhance quality of care and quality of life, a point neatly encapsulated by Evans:

> It is through our repeated experiences with patients that we begin to perceive the particular rather than the typical; care becomes individualised rather than standardised and planning becomes anticipatory of change rather than simply responsive to change.
>
> (Evans 1996: 15)

Nonetheless it is likely that the benefits of a stable workforce will not be fully realized in the absence of regular training and clinical supervision. In particular, unqualified staff need access to education which encourages them to value the older person's individuality and unique contribution to the life of the home. Stability among the staff of a home is likely to be enhanced by the introduction of a career structure for care assistants and the development of senior care assistant roles is already taking place within some homes, although systematic evaluation of such roles is limited. Such initiatives are likely to proliferate as the recommendations of the most recent strategy for nursing (Department of Health 1999c) come into effect. In particular, the proposal for more flexible programmes of nurse education and training are likely to encourage more care assistants to study for vocational qualifications.

Collectively, the evidence reviewed here suggests that we need to develop new cultures of care within care homes, which involve and value older people and their families, as well as valuing the providers of care (Nolan and Keady 1996). Willis and Linwood (1984) for example contrast the medical and holistic models of care prevalent within services for older people, with what they term the emancipatory model of care. This model assumes a horizontal relationship between the care provider and the older person and their family, with the role of the care provider being a supportive one. The emphasis is on interpersonal relationships and achieving a balance between preventive, curative and restorative care in full consultation with the older person. In a powerful paper on the challenges of older people's right to participation in health care, Walker (1999) also argues for change in professional values and attitudes within the formal sector so that cooperation and partnership with service users is seen as a normal activity.

At the beginning of the twenty-first century, no older person living in a care home should be subject to the 'personalized warehousing' approach to care first described so vividly by Miller and Gwynne in 1972, yet still so prevalent in many care homes today. It is no longer acceptable for any resident to merely have their physical needs met, particularly when the potential for enhancing quality of life through simple interventions is so enormous.

Bowsher (1994) suggests that the aims of long-term care should include older people being able to

- continue to develop competencies in new and different ways
- contribute to the development and maintenance of positive social support networks and social climates within their own social groups and nursing facility
- attain from their environment some of the things that are important or valued by them
- maintain some degree of congruence between desired and achieved goals
- experience satisfactions and positive affects even in their frailty
- generate some stories to tell about this time of their lives that are as interesting as those of their younger years.

Achieving these objectives, even with the most frail older person, should not be beyond our resources or wit.

6

Palliative care and older people

Jane E. Seymour and Elizabeth Hanson

One of the most significant social changes in the past 100 years has been the exponential growth in the proportion of older people and the heavy concentration of death at this stage of life. Although for many people old age is a period of independence and good health, for an increasing number it is associated with chronic, life-limiting illness and reduced resources for self-care. Death now occurs typically at the end of a long experience of old age. At the same time the ability or willingness of families to care for older people, and the adequacy of health and social care for both older people and their carers, are being questioned. The palliative care needs of these groups and the education of practitioners to meet them are thus of special significance if appropriate health and social services are to be developed.

Ley (1989), commenting on palliative care in gerontology, makes the fundamental point that palliative care is a philosophy: it is not necessarily associated with a particular setting, disease or type of caregiver. In spite of historical associations with cancer and hospices, palliative care is being recognized increasingly as essential for all those who are affected by, or suffer from, any life-threatening illness. Clark and Seymour (1999: 83) define the elements of palliative care as 'total care', referring to the multi-dimensional relief of the suffering of the ill person or their companions; 'teamwork', a model of interdisciplinary working required for effective holistic care; and 'trust' between the cared-for person and the caregivers, creating a relationship in which mutual autonomy is facilitated. The widely accepted definition of palliative care (World Health Organisation 1990) is predicated upon these principles, with the main aims being to

- affirm life and regard dying as a natural process
- neither hasten nor postpone death

- provide relief from pain and other distressing symptoms
- integrate the psychological and spiritual aspects of a patient care
- offer a support system to help the family cope during the patient's illness and their own bereavement.

(World Health Organisation 1990)

This chapter provides a brief historical overview of palliative care and gerontology, and then examines four key themes from a review of the literature in these fields:

- palliative care needs among older people: survey evidence
- palliative care provision for older people: the policy context
- living with palliative care needs: experiences of older people and their informal carers
- facing death: end-of-life decision making and older people.

New data from a series of in-depth interviews illuminate the discussion, particularly of the third theme, providing a sense of the personal experience of serious illness, disability and dying for older people and their family carers. Attention is focused on older people with non-cancer disease, a population especially disadvantaged in terms of their receipt of palliative care services. We conclude by making suggestions with regard to how palliative focused health care could be accessed more readily by all older people and their family carers.

A note about methodology

'Cross-Roads Care' in Sheffield identified a small group of nine chronically ill, heavily dependent older people and their nine family carers by mailing an anonymous request to participants in the study on our behalf. Those who felt able to contribute returned a pre-paid response to the authors, who then arranged appointments for interviews over the telephone. Prior to each interview fully informed and, where possible, written consent was obtained with participants being assured of confidentiality and anonymity. Consent was checked frequently throughout the dialogue following the principle of process consent (Usher and Arthur 1998; Seymour and Ingleton 1999).

Each of the ill participants either had suffered a stroke or had uncontrolled Parkinson's disease. They received care from the social services, and had intermittent and irregular contact with their primary health care team. Only one participant had experience of specialist palliative care services. While it is difficult to predict the remaining length of life for these individuals, studies suggest that in many cases they would be approaching the last year of their lives and have complex problems and symptoms which would be likely to benefit from specialist palliative care (Wilkinson *et al.* 1997; Addington-Hall *et al.* 1998a, b; Grande *et al.* 1998). Specialist palliative care is defined as:

those services with palliative care as their core speciality. They are delivered by professional staff with specialist training. Specialist palliative care teams are multidisciplinary and related to both general and hospital practice, being available to provide advice and support that bridges the divide between home and hospital and to provide hospice care. Education, research, and support of other health care professionals giving care with a palliative care approach are key roles for specialist palliative care.

(Clark and Seymour 1999: 86)

Specialist palliative care comprises four levels of intervention, ranging from advice and information to professional colleagues (for example, the primary health care team) but without direct patient contact; to close involvement in the ongoing assessment and clinical care of the patient and their family. Specialist palliative care practitioners may be nurses, doctors, social workers or psychologists, with provision being a multidisciplinary enterprise crossing institutional and agency boundaries.

Participants were asked about their daily lives, their health problems, the services they received, and what they thought would happen in the future. This latter question was worded carefully in an attempt to elicit some preferences regarding end-of-life care. What constituted 'good' and 'bad' care, and the personal and professional qualities which contributed to 'good' caring were explored. Interviews lasted on average for one hour: in some cases, a return visit was made to ensure that participants did not become too tired during what were potentially lengthy interviews.

While our research participants may be regarded as 'experts' in the identification of their care needs, their views are necessarily bounded within their own particular personal circumstances and cannot be taken as representative of all such individuals. Neither can they draw attention to the broader policy context within which their experiences of service delivery are largely fashioned. For these reasons we set their rich personal accounts in the context of the wider research and policy literature.

Palliative care and gerontology: common roots, divergent development

There is growing recognition that *all* people with longer term health and social care needs, irrespective of condition, should receive the benefits of palliative care (Gammon 1995; Hanrahan and Luchins 1995). However, the financial implications of this are huge. For example, Addington-Hall *et al.* (1998b) predicted an increase in specialist palliative care caseload of at least 79 per cent if such services were to be made fully available to those with non-cancer conditions. Whether we look at cancer or non-cancer disease, in almost all cases those needing palliative care are older. Cancer has a strikingly higher incidence among older people, particularly those aged

85 plus (Cleary and Carbone 1997); the incidence of life-limiting diseases such as chronic obstructive airways disease, circulatory disorders and Alzheimer's disease is weighted heavily towards older age groups. These latter conditions have an impact on patient and carer quality of life which is comparable to that experienced by the most severely affected cancer sufferers (Mogielnicki *et al.* 1990; Addington-Hall *et al.* 1995; Lynn *et al.* 1997; Addington-Hall *et al.* 1998a, b).

One of the strongest arguments for making palliative care services available to older people comes from the founder of the hospice movement, Dame Cicely Saunders, who always made it clear that her 'vision' included the care of older people: 'terminal care should not be a facet of oncology, but of geriatric medicine, neurology, general practice and throughout medicine' (Saunders and Baines 1983: 2). Indeed, it can be argued that modern palliative and hospice care share common foundations with gerontological medicine and nursing. Both developed in the early post-Second World War period against the backdrop of the new NHS with its overwhelmingly popular aim of caring for all in need from 'the cradle to the grave'. Public concern about the poor conditions in which ill and older people were cared for had been heightened by a series of state commissioned surveys conducted for pre-NHS implementation purposes (see for example Ministry of Health 1945); while surveys following in the wake of the influential Rowntree report of 1947 (Rowntree 1947) heightened awareness of the poverty and deprivation within the homes of many older people and their families. Sheldon's (1948) survey of Wolverhampton is perhaps the most famous of these. At the same time, concerns about the care of people of all ages who were dying were heightened as a result of surveys commissioned by newly formed charities (Marie Curie Memorial Foundation 1952; Glyn-Hughes 1960). During the same time period, Exton-Smith (1961) looked specifically at the problems associated with death in old age in a study of 220 dying older patients (Clark and Seymour 1999).

Geriatrics and palliative care, from their earliest days, have embraced a set of strikingly similar concerns. Both attend to the pursuit of symptom control, while advising the judicious use of investigations and rejecting highly invasive and aggressive treatment modalities; both make the person and their family the unit of care, and have led the way in developing multidisciplinary and community-based models of care. In so doing they have developed parallel discourses of 'patient-centred' care, 'quality of life', 'dignity' and 'autonomy'. Further, both disciplines focus on areas – ageing and cancer – that tend to provoke strong, even 'phobic' reactions from the public at large (Mount 1989).

Notwithstanding these similarities in philosophy, very different circumstances attend the delivery and experience of care within the two areas (Ahmedzai 1995; James and Field 1996; George and Sykes 1997), in spite of a policy of inclusion adopted by the hospice and palliative care movement (Standing Medical Advisory Committee (SMAC) and Standing

Nursing and Midwifery Advisory Committee (SNMAC) 1992). Access to high quality palliative care services seems to be dictated by local context (Bosanquet 1997) and the extent to which service providers have been able to overcome significant and structurally rooted 'disincentives to co-ordination, co-operation and communication' (Clark and Seymour 1999: 95). Indeed, palliative care has been marked by what Field (1994: 61) refers to as ' "five star" care for the select few', and has been able to rely on generous charitable donations and state support in its establishment of the hospice model for cancer sufferers. Partly as a result of this, but also due to the charismatic leadership of early hospice founders, hospice and palliative care have become emblematic of 'good death' – a central point of reference for popular expectations of dying and standards of care at the end of life (Clark and Seymour 1999). In contrast, those in receipt of gerontological care have been markedly disadvantaged (Cartwright *et al.* 1973; Cartwright 1993; Seale and Cartwright 1994) in terms of quality, quantity and coordination of care. One aspect of this disadvantage is the long-standing government policy of social exclusion in which services for older people have been seen as 'fair game' for cuts, means testing and shrinkage in state provision. This state-led policy of exclusion reinforces a wider public tendency to regard older people as 'socially dead' (Sudnow 1967; Mulkay 1993; Sweeting and Gilhoolhy 1997): perhaps less worthy of emotional and economic investment during their journey towards death. The wide-scale acceptance of the 'myth' of the burden of dependency (Warnes 1998) posed by older people feeds these socially exclusive practices and attitudes with the death of the 'too old' being an icon of the modern 'bad death'. Ahmedzai (1995) goes so far as to suggest that dying in old age is, in contemporary society, constituted by an 'epidemic of terminal suffering'.

We turn now to an analysis of evidence from large-scale surveys to explore palliative care needs among older people, before examining how patterns of palliative care provision are influenced by the wider policy context of service delivery, and translated into the personal experience of daily life for seriously ill older people and their family carers.

Palliative care needs among older people: survey evidence

Our understanding of patterns of dying and death among older people in the UK, and the prevalence of palliative care needs among this population, is informed largely by national interview surveys of those close to the deceased person during the last year of their life. These studies are concerned principally with the demographic profile and social circumstances of people during this period, their receipt of health and social care services and the incidence of pain and other symptoms. Cartwright *et al.* (1973) provided a framework that has since been replicated by Seale and

Cartwright (1994) and by Addington-Hall and McCarthy (1995). The problems inherent in proxy accounts thrown up by these studies are counterbalanced by the ethical and pragmatic difficulties of gaining the views of seriously ill persons in the last year of life (Cartwright and Seale 1990; Addington-Hall and McCarthy 1995).

Cartwright *et al.* (1973) explored the characteristics of random sample of all deaths which had occurred during a one-year period in 40 areas of England and Wales. Their aim was to develop a profile of care delivery with a focus on the use of formal and informal services. They revealed a range of problems:

- a lack of service coordination
- communication problems between service providers
- a dearth of practical, emotional and social support for informal carers who provide the majority of care.

Seale and Cartwright (1994) replicated this study, interviewing the bereaved companions or relatives of a sample of 800 people who had died during 12 months in 10 areas of England, while Addington-Hall and McCarthy (1995) surveyed 4000 companions of a random sample of people who died in 20 areas of the UK.

Seale and Cartwright (1994) demonstrated that older people in their sample were more likely to be women, less likely to be married and less likely to have living siblings to provide care. People aged 85 years and older were especially disadvantaged in terms of family support, but did not receive more attention from general practitioners or community nurses, even though they were least likely to be admitted to a hospital or hospice. In contrast, among the 65–85 cohort, the majority of deaths occurred within hospitals, in spite of the acknowledged preference among the majority of older people to remain at home (Hinton 1979; Wilkes 1984; Townsend *et al.* 1990). Overall, Seale and Cartwright (1994) calculate that 22 per cent of 'bed days' are used by those in the last year of their lives, and that the majority of these are from older age groups.

These trends were particularly prevalent among older people who died from non-cancer disease. They suffered longer periods of dependency and illness than cancer sufferers, and received care that was comparatively poorly coordinated. Seale and Cartwright (1994: 87) concluded that such individuals are 'relatively neglected in relation to care and research', with the 'lack of responsiveness of the medical and nursing services to the needs of older people in the last year of their lives' being an indication of a law of 'inverse care' (Seale and Cartwright 1994).

Addington-Hall and McCarthy (1995) examined the prevalence of physical symptoms and pain among dying people and the type of services they received, publishing valuable information about the circumstances of people dying from cancer, stroke (Addington-Hall *et al.* 1995, 1998a) and dementia (McCarthy *et al.* 1997). In a detailed comparison of cancer and non-cancer deaths, Addington-Hall *et al.* (1998b) concluded that one in six non-cancer patients experience symptom loads which are similar to the most severely affected cancer patients, but that specialist palliative care services are almost exclusively delivered to those with cancer. Extrapolating from their data they argue that approximately 71,744 people who die from non-malignant disease in England and Wales each year have specialist palliative care needs, and that this group are, on average, older than those with similar levels of need in the cancer population.

Palliative care provision for older people: the policy context

From the above it is clear that older people with palliative care needs are less well served than their younger counterparts. Both the Audit Commission (1997) report and the Clinical Standards Advisory Group (CSAG 1998) report on community care highlight a 'vicious circle' so that responsibility for older people tends to fall between health and social care agencies. The redefinition of 'health' as 'social' need during old age, and the consequent erosion in state provision may represent the greatest barrier to the development of integrated palliative care provision for older people (Clark and Seymour 1999: 97).

Most recently, the Royal Commission on Long-Term Care (1999) reported major shortcomings in service provision and financial arrangements for frail and ill older people in need of care and support. Many older people with palliative care needs find themselves having to pay for nursing and personal care either within institutional settings or their own homes, which others receive free purely by dint of differing diagnosis and age:

> Whereas the state through the NHS pays for all the care needs of sufferers from, for example cancer and heart disease, people who suffer from Alzheimer's disease may get little or no help with the cost of comparable care needs. All these conditions are debilitating, but Alzheimer's disease cannot yet be cured by medical intervention. However, a mixture of all types of care, including personal care will be needed. This is directly analogous to the kind of care provided for cancer sufferers. The latter get their care free. The former have to pay.
> (Royal Commission on Long-Term Care 1999: ch. 4)

The Royal Commission on Long-Term Care (1999) thus highlights a system of health and social care which is 'characterized by complexity and unfairness in the way it operates' and which 'contains a number of providers and funders of care, each of whom has different management or financial interests which may work against the interests of the individual client'. As a result, for many older people, care is less focused on rehabilitation, quality of life and the promotion of independence – all key elements of good palliative and gerontological care – and more concerned with the limitation of the short-term costs incurred by the local providers of care. As a consequence, preventive and assessment strategies are poorly developed and 'crisis' intervention becomes the norm during the illnesses of old age.

Arising from this process of 'cost-shunting' from health care (which remains free at the point of delivery), to social care (which is means-tested) has been a proliferation of private care homes. The number of NHS long-stay beds has reduced by 38 per cent since 1983 (a loss of 21,300 beds), and the number of private nursing home places has increased by 900 per cent (an increase of 141,000 beds) (Royal Commission 1999). As the Royal Commission noted, in the late twentieth century it was common for frail older people:

> often upon discharge from hospital, or from their own homes, often in a crisis, to go into residential or nursing homes. As a result they are forced to sell their homes, sever their links with their local community and end their days in settings which are usually caring and supportive, but which in some senses remove older people from our sight and from society at large. Individuals then suffer social exclusion; society colludes in this by too often regarding older people in these settings as being not only out of sight but also out of mind.
> (Royal Commission on Long-Term Care 1999: ch. 1)

Two elements appear to have contributed to this growth of private care homes. First, the limited capacity within the acute care sector of the NHS to cater for the needs of older people who may take longer to recuperate or who may linger longer during the dying phase of a long-term chronic illness. Second, the availability of social security payments for long-term care, although private individuals still bear much of the cost for such care.

It is against this background that the needs of older people requiring palliative care should be considered. We turn now to an examination of the experience of living with palliative care needs for older people and their informal carers, focusing in particular on the situation of those in receipt of 'community care' whether at home or in institutional care.

Living with palliative care needs: experiences of older people and their informal carers

Community care and family care giving

Respondents in our small-scale study stated repeatedly that they often felt 'abandoned' by the health care system which focuses mainly on particular clinical tasks or on crisis intervention. Comments such as 'they don't get in contact with me unless I ring them for some reason' were prevalent in the interviews, echoing similar recent observations on the care and services received by people suffering from Chronic Obstructive Pulmonary Disease (Skilbeck *et al.* 1998; Rhodes and Shaw 1999). Assessment of care needs and ongoing evaluation or planning for future needs were conspicuously absent, as described by one of the participants in our study, when speaking of his experience of respite care:

> Well perhaps the first thing that would have to be done would be to get the old person and assess the situation of the patient, and that would be a delicate process according to the response from the patient . . . The first person that visited knew what our role was but has never been since [coordinator of respite care service] and it was never enquired of me how it's going on – that's almost a criticism, [but] that's probably a requirement that someone in charge has to say 'is that position going through fine – what is happening?'
>
> (Interview 1)

A sense of therapeutic nihilism was also apparent with many participants remembering health care professionals stating 'there is nothing more we can do'. One older woman described vividly how she and her husband, who had a dense right hemi-plegia, felt upset and angry when physiotherapy had been discontinued after his discharge home, in spite of their perception that this would have been beneficial. The feelings that this sort of experience engendered were voiced by another severely disabled older man:

> I've had therapy and [now] they've pushed me to one side.
>
> (Interview 2)

In consequence a diminished sense of social worth permeated these interviews, with participants expressing fears of what would happen if their condition deteriorated or if their carer become infirm and unable to continue to care for them at home. The phrase 'if we can just carry on as we are' was mentioned frequently by almost all the respondents.

All the older people in our sample shared a situation of dependency and marginalization regardless of whether they were the givers or receivers of care. Carers generally felt neglected in terms of the amount and continuity of support they received, although their contact with particular individuals was usually reported favourably. Isolation, a fervent desire to carry on 'coping', coupled with a sense of having to muddle through with support that was barely adequate, often unsuitable and difficult to find out about, was prevalent:

> seeking help, and the help being there, knowing it is, that's one of the problems of any big city, you don't know how good somebody is, somebody might have an excellent service at that end of the city – again the problem is there doesn't seem one place to start. To me it is not coordinated, there's social service, when I enquire about

something for the bathroom they put me onto a place opposite [name of another office], and then your doctor will say I'll put you on to so and so.

(Interview 1)

This same respondent, a man in his mid-eighties, gave an insight into his feelings about caring for his much loved wife of 59 years who had suffered a stroke and was now showing signs of advanced dementia. Of particular note in his account was a perhaps paradoxical sense of loneliness combined with an unwillingness to accept care that he deemed inappropriate for his and his wife's needs. Explaining this paradox, he described how he felt that the 'delicate process' of developing a rapport with his wife had not been engaged with by outside carers. He felt they were insensitive to his wife's needs and therefore found it difficult to entrust her care to them. His comments on the waxing and waning of hope in his life are especially poignant:

I hope she and I are able to stay together. But of course in the back of my mind is that she will eventually get worse and have to go into a home, that's facing up to the situation isn't it . . . there isn't any hope, you see, this is the awful realization that this is the end of the road. Nobody can help you really can they?

(Interview 1)

As this older man fears, the likelihood of his wife ending her days in institutional care is high. Indeed, age cohort appears to be a key determinant of the setting within which older people tend to receive care at the end of their lives and where they die (Grande *et al.* 1998).

Institutional care

Approximately 25 per cent of all older people aged 85 years and over live in residential and nursing homes (House of Commons Health Committee 1996; Royal Commission on Long-Term Care 1999) and 15 per cent of all deaths now occur in such settings (Bury and Holme 1991; Seale and Cartwright 1994; Clark and Seymour 1999). Those who enter institutional care tend to have greater physical and mental frailty than those who live at home, a poorer quality of life, and to be more socially isolated (Seale and Cartwright 1994). Despite these complex needs, there are acute shortages of both trained and untrained staff and limited availability of the specialist equipment needed for appropriate palliative care (Siddell *et al.* 1998). A widespread lack of education and understanding of palliative care issues, together with a sense of isolation among home care staff, exacerbate such resource issues. Siddell *et al.* (1998) note that while care staff are willing to care for residents until death and are motivated to provide a high standard of care, resource constraints and a lack of investment from the wider community means that dying in such establishments remains 'a scandal waiting to happen' (Royal College of Nursing 1992).

Medical responsibility for residents' care is of special note, and currently falls 'by default rather than design upon the heavily burdened shoulders of the general practitioner' (Black and Bowman 1997), a situation which is inimical to the proactive clinical strategies necessary for effective pain and symptom relief. As Katz *et al.* (1999) conclude, this situation has led to isolation and inadequate care delivery in many homes.

Not surprisingly then, anxiety and worry about the entry to care pervaded our respondents' accounts: an issue highlighted as being of particular significance in earlier work by Nolan *et al.* (1996a). The term 'putting away' was used frequently by our participants:

> I don't want to let go, I want to do it all, but I've got to face [it] – inevitably she will deteriorate and then will come the trauma of putting her away.
>
> (Interview 1)

It was difficult to glean how most disabled participants felt about care home entry. In most cases this was because of speech impairment. In some cases, they made wry faces when respite care was mentioned, or raised their eyebrows to express distaste or unhappiness. Others communicated their fears about respite care very effectively:

> *Wife:* . . . he goes into respite sometimes, but he doesn't like it.
> *Interviewer:* You prefer to be at home, Mr X?
> *Husband:* No, respite. Oh no. Oh no, no, no, – Oh Christ, respite, oh no, no, no.
> *Wife:* All right then you're not going.
> *Husband:* Hoist, hoist.
> *Wife:* It's the hoist, they don't lift him properly. They don't lift you properly [do they]?
>
> (Interview 4)

Another respondent who had unstable epilepsy described his fears of being left unattended and possibly dying while in respite care:

> *Husband:* . . . I go into respite care every eight weeks for two weeks and I'm due on the 30th March . . . It gives [wife] a rest, she can do what she likes.
> *Interviewer:* So you don't mind going?
> *Husband:* No. Only thing wrong is pressing these buzzers and they're sometimes about ten minutes coming. Well, if I start – I can be out before they come.
>
> (Interview 3)

These fears meant that his wife was keen to minimize his entry to care whenever she could:

Wife: If I could manage and I had my way he wouldn't go into respite at all, I'd prefer him to be at home.

(Interview 3)

In contrast, another man in his early seventies with severe unstable Parkinson's disease reported positive experiences of respite care in a local hospice. His greatest regret was, however, that he was not able to receive such care for more than two weeks in every six months.

So far, we have addressed the daily lives of older people with palliative care needs and their carers and their feelings about institutional care. However, an important part of palliative care is the management of the terminal phase of illness, when questions about place of death and end-of-life decision making become critical. It is to this period that we now turn.

Facing death: end-of-life decision making and older people

The issue of autonomy has become pre-eminent in discussions about end-of-life care. Autonomy, on which the legal right of informed consent is based, is the capacity for self-determination and choice, free both from exterior compulsion or internal impairment (Pabst-Battin 1994). The exploration of 'autonomous' preferences for care at the end of life, and the management of clinical decisions informed by such preferences, can be extremely complex in the case of older people. Greater diagnostic uncertainty makes it difficult to predict 'dying' accurately; this affects the degree to which patients are aware of their lives being limited, and the extent to which clinicians can begin to shift their emphasis to palliative, rather than curative, care. Further, the diagnosis of dying in older people may often be made only by exclusion (Blackburn 1989), leaving little time for the careful and compassionate communications between patient, family and health care staff on which good 'person-centred' palliative care depends. Diagnostic difficulty is compounded frequently by mental disorder and severe disability, which makes ascertaining older people's preferences a considerable challenge (Graham and Livesley 1983; Blackburn 1989; Dunstan 1996). A central issue in most debates about end-of-life care concerns 'personhood' and the extent to which the essence of personhood and preferences change during the course of the bodily deterioration associated with illness.

The ethical, moral and clinical problems associated with individual patients who can no longer express preferences are compounded by the recognition that individual treatment decisions are constrained and influenced by wider economic and social factors. This recognition gives rise to fears of a rapid slide down a 'slippery slope' (Keown 1995) if there is any relaxation of the laws regarding end of life care. In all their forms, 'slippery slope' arguments against the legalization of euthanasia or physician-assisted suicide point to the possible pre-eminence of such factors in end-of-life decision making, leading to discrimination against those who are considered to be an economic or social burden. Recent examples of such fears are the reports in the popular press during December 1999 of 'euthanasia by the back door' in the UK for some older people and signs that the decriminalization of voluntary euthanasia in the Netherlands has resulted in cases of 'involuntary euthanasia' in older people with Alzheimer's disease and other conditions in that country (Keown 1995).

Further, these arguments apply not only to the situation of those older people who have lost the ability to express their wishes and needs, but also to those who can make their choices known (Howse 1998). A powerful argument against the legalization of voluntary euthanasia has come from those who point to the risk of coerced altruism becoming a significant element in such requests as a result of the ideological power of polemics which defend health care rationing on the basis of age (Callahan 1987). Smith (1994) in a letter responding to an assertion from the Netherlands that euthanasia can be part of 'good palliative care' (Heintz 1994) highlights the existence of this theme in the thinking behind the rejection of legalized voluntary euthanasia by the House of Lords Select Committee on Medical Ethics. Many in the palliative care and hospice movement (National Council for Hospice and Specialist Palliative Care Services (NCHSPCS) 1993; Sachs *et al.* 1995; Twycross 1995; NCHSPCS 1997) argue that euthanasia may become an easy alternative to the greater challenge of addressing problems regarding care delivery and planning for those groups of vulnerable people who have been described as the 'disadvantaged' dying (Harris 1990).

Moreover, requests for euthanasia may not be the result of 'rational' autonomous deliberation but rather depression among physically ill older people (Lindesay 1991). Findings from Chochinov *et al.* (1995) showed that of 200 terminally ill people they interviewed, only 8.5 per cent had a 'serious and pervasive wish to die', and that this was associated significantly with measures of depression. However, an epidemiological study by Jorm *et al.* (1995) revealed that when the influence of depression was controlled, poor self-rated health, disability, hearing and visual impairment, living in residential care and not being married were important risk factors in the wish to die in older people. Of these, the strongest association was with residential care.

Seale and Addington-Hall (1994), using interview data from their large-scale survey of bereaved people, have shown that requests for euthanasia by dying people, and beliefs on the part of bereaved people that an earlier death would have been preferable for their companions, are associated with high levels of dependency and those 'symptoms particularly associated with very old age, such as loss of bladder and bowel control and mental confusion' (Seale and Addington-Hall 1994: 654). In a related paper examining the views of dying people and their companions about the best time to die, Seale and Addington-Hall (1995) conclude that very elderly people, particularly women, are much more likely to be reported as saying that they wanted to die sooner.

While it was difficult to examine such issues directly with our respondents, we have some evidence that supports the foregoing arguments. One respondent was particularly blunt when asked what his thoughts were about the present and the future:

> R: I watch telly and I count the bricks on the wall . . . that's all I do. Sit here. . . . I think about snuffing it.
>
> I: Do you?
>
> R: Oh aye, because that's all I'm worth, isn't it? 85 years old. Well, it's where we all end isn't it? We all end up in the same place, don't we?
>
> I: Does it worry you?
>
> R: It worries me a little bit, but I can't avoid it, so I don't let it worry me too much.
>
> (Interview 2)

The wider literature suggests that older people wish to influence the timing, manner and circumstances of their own deaths, while rejecting active euthanasia or physician-assisted suicide (Kelner 1995). Such research is important, given the relative infrequency with which older people complete advance directives and evidence that clinicians and the legal profession are more likely to disregard preferences expressed by people from disadvantaged social groups (Morrow 1997). Key themes from studies exploring end-of-life issues with older people (Cohen-Mansfield *et al.* 1991; Gamble *et al.* 1991; Kellogg *et al.* 1992; Heap *et al.* 1993; Liddle *et al.* 1993; Kelner 1995) are:

- Older people welcome the opportunity to discuss end-of-life issues and the majority would wish to have such a discussion with their professional care staff.
- Anxieties are present among older people that possession of a 'living will' may lead to the premature withdrawal of treatment by clinicians.
- The language of advance treatment directives is poorly understood: many older people with such directives would still choose to be resuscitated.
- Preference for non-treatment tends to be associated with the permanence of the treatment proposed, and perceptions of poor prognosis and impaired cognitive function rather than with age or any other socio-demographic variable.
- Older people often have a preferred 'proxy' but frequently have not discussed their care preferences with that individual.
- Older people make assumptions that their family members will reach a consensus decision about their end-of-life care.

Our data suggest that the latter two points about families acting as advocates are of critical importance. Carer participants often feared becoming ill themselves, partly because this would lead to an admission into care for their spouse, and partly because they were aware that they had a responsibility for representing the wants and interests of their spouse. Anxieties were often tied up with previous bad experiences and worries about wider family obligations:

> I worry about what would happen to [husband] if anything happened to me, because I think that Social Services run circles round him, and that rather concerns me. Because one person, I can't remember which one it was that came from Social Services, and I said something about paying for care, if he had to go into care. 'Well you've got this beautiful bungalow' [they said]. I said, 'I'm sorry, but half of this bungalow belongs to my daughters.' But they had already, in the back of their minds, got the idea that there was a bungalow that they could draw on to keep [husband] in care if anything happened to me.
>
> (Interview 6)

The caring professions and palliative care for all: ways forward?

The National Council for Hospice and Specialist Palliative Care Services (Addington-Hall 1998) has recognized the need to extend palliative care to all those in need, regardless of diagnosis, or personal resources. Innovative partnerships between statutory and voluntary services, the development of care pathways, and the introduction of joint appointments in palliative care which cross-sector boundaries are seen as essential to developing a culture of integration and collaboration (Black and Bowman 1997). Clark and Seymour (1999) summarize the recommendations of a range of sources that suggest the necessary requirements for progress to be made:

- abolishing the division between residential and nursing homes, and developing a spectrum of homes serving different needs
- placing registration of homes with a National Office for Standards of Care
- developing a comprehensive assessment tool covering health and social needs to ensure the appropriate placement of older people
- introducing specialist nurses to ensure adequate assessment and supervision of care standards.

Rhodes and Shaw (1999) suggest that policy documents such as the White Paper, *The New NHS* (Department of Health 1997a) are likely to have a positive effect on palliative care services because they emphasize active partnerships between all agencies. Such an explicit emphasis promises more effective coordination of services for people living in the community. Further, the renewed focus on the role of professional community care staff in conducting comprehensive assessments and monitoring of needs of older people and their family carers has the potential to improve the situation of all those who are affected by serious life-limiting illness (Daniels 1999; Morris and Bowman 1999). One of our participants and his wife highlighted vividly the need for such an approach when they were asked about the formal services they received:

> I feel we've had to be very proactive to get it (care, equipment and supplies) – no one takes overall responsibility – each of the professionals assume that I am being taken care of somewhere else – whether it's the district nurse for catheter care or the Parkinson's disease nurse about my illness – everyone sees to every little bit – [but] there's no one who just looks after the people.
>
> (Interview 9)

A pilot evaluation study has suggested that providing specialist community palliative care support to nursing homes helps to bridge the barriers between statutory health services and the private sector both by overcoming nursing home isolation and improving equity of access to specialist palliative care (Avis *et al.* 1999). In our local area, a Macmillan nurse team operating from a hospice has initiated liaison with nursing homes using funds previously used exclusively for hospices. This, it is felt, has led to higher standards of palliative care delivery among care staff by improving knowledge, resources and recognition of this aspect of care. This liaison service has placed emphasis upon, first, the importance of 'simple' things which often have huge benefits in terms of an individual's quality of life, and second, team discussion about a person's needs and the most appropriate and realistic way of addressing them (personal communication).

Such a person-centred approach based upon individual need is pivotal to the delivery of good palliative care. For example Corner and Dunlop (1997) argue that a person's emotional experience is inseparable from their physical experience and urge a 'reframing of care' to encompass a meaning centred approach in which 'the individual and their own understanding is placed at the core of therapeutic intervention' (Corner and Dunlop 1997: 300). Bycock (1996) emphasizes the potential for developing therapeutic strategies to relieve suffering and enable 'the person to attain a sense of completion within the social and interpersonal dimensions, [and] to develop or deepen a sense of worthiness and to find their own unique sense of meaning of life' (Bycock 1996: 251).

Echoing a similar philosophy, the work of Kitwood (see for example Kitwood 1993, 1997) in dementia highlights practical approaches to enhancing personhood and dignity even in the face of profound cognitive impairment and bodily dissolution. Kitwood argues that concepts of 'personhood' and 'dignity' flow between people and are invested in the *manner* in which care is given. Thus, personhood, on which well-being and dignity depend, is essentially social: it is not determined by intactness

of 'self', but rather is vested in relationships between people. Our participants confirmed that the intersubjective enhancement of personhood
through the sensitive delivery of 'basic' care is possible. Detailed descriptions from several participants about care workers whom they regarded as
experts, indicated that these care workers were 'in tune' with their own
personal ways of 'doing' or 'being' – qualities which were most evident
during the delivery of potentially difficult or embarrassing intimate care:

> At morning and dressing, N [care worker] knows everything to do
> now. John's a man of habit and he likes to do things just as he wants.
> N knows exactly what John likes and we've no problems there.
>
> (Interview 3)

Participants spoke about the personal qualities of the care worker that suggested they respected and knew the older person as a person. In such cases
they enjoyed their time with the worker, and had become friends. A sense
of reciprocal giving and receiving of friendship emerged which enhanced
participants' feeling of social worth:

> Well, I think they care – I don't think they come in because they think
> they have to – I think they think it's a pleasure to come – they all give
> us that impression, and they're kind to him and to me as well.
>
> (Interview 2)

> Well, it's his attitude towards John. He doesn't try and rush him. He
> knows exactly what to do, he doesn't hassle him, he just lets him take
> his time. We've got to more like friends now, haven't we?
>
> (Interview 3)

Sometimes, carers hinted that verbal communication was not always
essential, rather a sense of 'being with' the person and understanding their
facial expression and body posture was highly valued:

> She's a very quiet girl – her approach is very good – she even under-
> stands what he says.
>
> (Interview 6)

This almost intangible skill of 'being with' the patient is highlighted
within the palliative care nursing literature as an integral part of the
nurse's empathic skills (Degner and Gow 1991; Davies *et al.* 1999; Hanson
and Culihall 1995), and is further highlighted in the wider literature in
Chapter 2.

The sensitive use of physical comfort and touch is a particularly important aspect of the delivery of care to dying and seriously ill people in whom
sense of hearing and sight may be failing (Morse *et al.* 1994). This was
highlighted by our carer respondents who gave vivid examples of situations in which professional carers handled their husband or wife roughly,
communicating both a lack of respect and a disregard for the dignity of
their spouse:

They want to be here and gone and they're in too much of a rush and pull him off balance, and then he gets irritable because he's not in control. Having had crushed kneecaps, when he tries to sit down, he's got to go down very carefully, and they put their hand on his shoulder and push him – Get down!

(Interview 6)

In contrast, examples were also provided in which careworkers assisted the person in a very different manner, communicating not only gentleness, but also security, safety and respect. The difference is often subtle, but nonetheless very real for those in receipt of such care or the watchful co-carer of the person:

She's gentle with him, she knows what he wants – And she's quiet when she says – come along Roy, move your weight to so and so please. And he'll move his weight and she'll get him where she wants without pushing. And she'll move him over very quietly without any pushing. Generally her attitude is more a concern for the patient than in getting a job done and getting out as quick as she can.

(Interview 6)

As well as sensitive approaches to physical care giving, biography and life history are increasingly being recognized as important when working with older people, particularly in long-term care settings, in order to understand their past and thus explore their hopes and aspirations for the future. Indeed Best (1998: 23) argues that without biographical understanding (perhaps through facilitating story-telling), care lacks a thorough foundation and carers may, albeit unwittingly, be 'negligent in the care [they] provide' (Best 1998: 23). However, continuity of care is essential to the successful facilitation of such approaches (Nolan *et al.* 1996a). Yet, for our respondents, change rather than continuity was the norm, and this was a fundamental barrier to the development of *any* relationship let alone one in which hopes and fears could be explored and mutual respect and dignity enhanced. One couple explained how many difficulties flowed from frequent changes in care staff, with time spent needlessly explaining how care was to be given, rather than in developing relationships and enhancing well-being:

Wife: Oh yes, this is the problem, you get somebody different every night.
Husband: Because when it's a different one that's never been, she's got a lot of explaining to do.
Wife: I have to start all over again what he needs doing for him and how to do it.

(Interview 3)

While the foregoing has concentrated on interpersonal skills and attributes of compassionate nursing care, there is also considerable evidence of the lack of the specialist palliative care clinical skills that are necessary for the adequate control of pain and other troublesome symptoms. Recent evidence suggests that some older people with non-cancer disease are profoundly disadvantaged in terms of symptom control. While cancer patients often experience a number of intensely distressing symptoms which have a rapid onset over a shorter period of time, those with non-cancer are more likely to have experienced similar symptoms for at least a year. Further, older people with chronic non-cancer disease are more likely to have been restricted in activities of daily living for a longer time period and to have experienced additional symptoms such as mental confusion, incontinence, difficulty hearing and seeing, and dizziness (Addington-Hall 1998).

Pain is a prevalent symptom for the majority of older people in the last year of life whether suffering from cancer or non-cancer (Addington-Hall *et al.* 1998a, b), and yet pain remains poorly recognized and under-treated (Aronheim 1997). In residential and nursing homes a lack of knowledge and skills regarding the assessment and management of both acute and chronic pain has long been acknowledged (Gibbs 1995; Maestri-Banks and Gosney 1997; Siddell *et al.* 1998), and seems to result from poor medical cover and a tendency not to refer patients to specialist palliative care services. The problem is compounded for those who cannot com-municate their pain to those caring for them. Lack of regular assessment using pain instruments, inappropriate or underuse of opioid analgesia, and an ignorance of non-pharmacological methods of pain management have all been identified (Parkes 1992; Ferrell and Ferrell 1993; Closs 1996).

The challenge is to make available specialist skills in hospice and palliative care to all older people whether living at home, in institutional care, or in hospital. As Saunders *et al.* (1981) stated, hospice is not a place, but rather a *concept* of care that embraces a range of approaches from the subtle skills of 'being with' someone to the most advanced modes of pharmacological symptom control. We must acknowledge the need for more effective educational preparation of professional carers working with older people in all settings and the value of a palliative care approach at an earlier stage of the illness trajectory. We also need to promote the value of prompt specialist advice with regard to pain and symptom control and closer collaboration between health and social care providers.

Conclusion

Writing about the care of older people with dementia in 1992, but expressing sentiments which apply to care for all older people, Kitwood and Bredin observed:

> thousands upon thousands of hours of care work pass by, in which the people involved generally do not understand what they are doing . . .

a care practice, however good it might be, is relatively ineffective
without a coherent theory: it is powerless at the clinical, pedagogical
and political levels. A thorough theorisation . . . provides awareness,
a sense of value, and the basis for concerted action.

(Kitwood and Bredin 1992a: 270)

Our review of the literature and small exploration of the palliative care
needs of older people and their carers suggest an urgent need for such
theorization if disadvantage and discrimination are to end. Palliative care,
it seems, must engage on a broadly political base with a 'moral order' of
suffering (Clark 1997), so that the experience of dying for older people is
seen as no less worthy than that of younger people. One of our participants spoke eloquently of facing a 'yawning chasm', saying that the challenge for nursing, and by implication for all the caring professions, was to
help him face a frightening future with a degree of hope.

The assumption that illness and death are somehow 'natural' for older
people, and that they 'disengage' from their lives with relative ease as
death approaches has to be challenged (Howarth 1998). Death, it is
believed, is easy for older people (Howarth 1998: 673) since their 'natural'
lifespan has come to an end, and there are no more reasons for living. This
perception is exacerbated by the pervasive tendency to view 'quality of
life' within a primarily functional framework. Nihilism and feelings of
hopelessness result for both professional staff and older people. Moreover,
this perspective denies the possibility, promoted by 'good death' ideologies, that dying can be a positive part of the life cycle in which opportunities arise to 'reintegrate' with life and to develop a heightened sense
of well-being (Bycock 1996).

The experience of not being able to achieve the high standards of 'good
death' inherent within the latter perspective may lead to a sense of failure
within health and social care professionals. Low pay, environmental,
social and economic constraints clearly coalesce to make this appear an
impossible goal within the realities of old age care as delivered currently.
The devaluation of caring work – always a theme in commentaries on
family care – is perpetuated by the low status, lack of appropriate education and training, and heavy responsibilities placed on care staff in the
different theatres of old age care, particularly those without professional
qualifications (Nolan and Keady 1996). Palliative focused care depends
upon the personal integrity of care staff being nurtured: it cannot be delivered in a situation of clear discrimination towards those engaged with the
'dirty' work that many people would rather not think about. Just as dignity and personhood depend on the quality of social interaction between
ill people and those caring for them, so the occupational and professional
integrity of care workers must be supported and promoted by institutional
structures, managerial cultures and social policies (de Raeve 1996).

A useful reformulation of the 'good death' concept has been put forward
by McNamara (1997) which suggests how the standards associated with

hospice style palliative care may be married with the realities impinging on the care of older people. The 'good enough death' recognizes the role of exterior constraints in moulding the context within which care is given and received, and allows for a more pragmatic and contingent conceptualization in which an inability to achieve all the highest standards within hospice and palliative care ideology becomes recognized as a reality rather than a failure. The 'good enough death' offers an opportunity to conceive of efforts to strive for a high standard of care as worthwhile in themselves, rather than a fruitless battle against impossible odds. What is needed, as Kitwood and Bredin (1992a) suggest, is a theoretical framework to identify and legitimize key aspects.

Good palliative care, whether delivered by specialist or non-specialist practitioners, is worth struggling for: we must all take up the challenge.

7

The mental health needs of older people and their carers: exploring tensions and new directions

Claire Ferguson and John Keady

In writing this chapter we faced a number of significant challenges arising primarily from the extensive but fragmented literature on the mental health needs of older people, a literature which encompasses a diverse range of subjects including the nature and meaning of mental health/illness/ageing; the demography and epidemiology of various conditions; subjective adaptation and adjustment to the onset and progression of illness; carer's needs; mental health care within community and residential settings; legal issues; health promotion; service response, assessment, intervention, training, organization and teamworking; service evaluation; societal attitudes and the enduring impact of ageism on the health and social care system; and the development, implementation and evaluation of local and national policy frameworks. Despite the breadth of the literature, coverage was peculiarly one-sided with an extensive consideration in some areas, such as dementia, and very little in others, for example, depression.

In developing a degree of conceptual order it was apparent that the literature could be considered under two main headings relating either to specific mental health needs, or to issues that transcended individual conditions and applied more generally, such as ethnicity or living arrangements. Within each of these areas, further subdivisions were possible, for example by focusing on issues of prevalence or practice and professional development. Much of the literature in this latter area was anecdotal, lacking adequate and rigorous empirical verification. Moreover, despite the rhetoric of involvement, the voices of users and carers were muted within the literature consulted. Such opinions appear largely invisible in the academic literature, expressing themselves in other vehicles such as Asylum and Open Mind.

Notwithstanding these limitations, the volume of literature was such that it is not possible to explore all avenues. Rather our aim in this chapter is to distil the major themes emerging from the literature and to consider their implications for developing services intended to enhance the quality of care and quality of life for older people and their carers. The chapter is primarily constructed around three core themes progressing from the more general policy context, via professional ideologies and finally to training. These themes unfold as follows:

- developing an integrated policy and service framework
- creating a new vision for professional assessment and intervention
- reconfiguring professional training and role identity.

In order to contextualize the review, the chapter begins by attending to a number of issues emerging from the epidemiological literature, as well as identifying some obvious areas where there has been little or no empirical or theoretical work.

Constructing the chapter: some personal observations and reflections

From the sociological literature it almost appears that dementia is taken as synonymous with mental illness in older age. This is not helped by the dearth of theoretical or empirical studies in other areas, for instance depression and its impact on family caring (see for example Badger 1996). This is quite surprising given that depression is the most prevalent mental health problem in older age. Inevitably therefore this chapter draws heavily on the literature on dementia. This should not be seen to reflect any personal bias on our part. It merely mirrors the available literature. Furthermore, in order to illustrate some of the implications for practice development we mainly use the nursing literature. This should not be construed as representing a unidisciplinary approach. It is also appropriate at this stage to raise potential tensions about the value of a separate consideration of mental health in older age. This, it could be argued, might perpetuate the exclusion of older people from mainstream mental health services and exacerbate rather than ameliorate negative attitudes (see Ashton and Keady 1999; Reed and Clarke 1999b). This is certainly not our intention. Rather we believe that it is necessary to explore further the experience of mental health provision in older age in order that better informed and more appropriate service responses might ensue. That is our aim in this chapter.

The mental health care of older people and their carers: establishing a context

Epidemiological considerations

Numerous conditions fall under the umbrella term of 'mental health/illness' in old age; these include dementia; depression and adjustment reactions; suicide; schizophrenia; substance misuse; delirium; and anxiety disorders (see World Health Organisation 1992; American Psychiatric Association 1994). In addition, many older people experience homelessness; HIV/AIDS; loneliness; poverty; economic vulnerability; war and displacement; and are the victims of elder and sexual abuse, experiences that are manifest both in the developed and developing world (for a discussion see Levkoff *et al.* 1995). Furthermore, in the UK the Department of Health (1997b) issued a *Handbook on the Mental Health of Older People* which (on page 26), highlighted additional areas potentially influencing the mental health of older people, particularly for those individuals:

* leaving institutions after many years
* with impaired vision and hearing
* from ethnic minority groups
* without carers
* with learning difficulties
* with physical disabilities and mobility problems.

Despite this diversity, a significant proportion of the literature focuses on the prevalence of mental health problems among older people/populations in nursing homes, or within 'geriatric' units. However, due to methodological problems, and differences in the populations studied, this work is often contradictory and confusing to interpret. Lawlor and Radic (1994) summarizes this succinctly, by stating that:

> mental illness is common in the elderly, but prevalence figures vary widely according to the populations surveyed and the methodologies used.
>
> (Lawlor and Radic 1994: 157)

Notwithstanding these limitations, the epidemiological literature is fairly clear that depression and dementia are among the most prevalent forms of mental health problems in old age, with HIV/AIDS, alcohol misuse, living arrangements and the needs of ethnic minority elders being among the most neglected. Therefore, the prevalence rates and some key points with respect to these conditions are briefly rehearsed in order to provide a context for the remainder of the review.

Dementia

According to Prince (1985) by 2000 the numbers of people aged 65 and over would be about 423 million world-wide, with nearly 50 per cent of this total living in developing countries. Prince (1985) further suggests that by 2025 there will be 34.1 million people with some form of dementia, 24.2 million in the developing countries and 9.9 million living in the developed world. In examining the situation in Europe, Hofman *et al.* (1991) conducted an extensive multi-method prevalence study (EURO-DEM) taking account of the detailed case analysis of samples of older people from twelve European countries. Investigating retrospective prevalence rates between 1980 and 1990, Hofman *et al.* (1991) detailed the age and gender-specific estimates of the prevalence of dementia using the *DSM-III-R* (American Psychiatric Association 1987) and *ICD-10* (World Health Organisation 1992) standard diagnostic tools as entry criteria for the study. Of the 12 participating countries – which included the UK (although only sites in England were chosen), Finland, Italy, Spain and Sweden among others – it was found that general age and gender distribution were similar for all countries, with the overall European prevalence of dementia for the five year age groups from 60 to 94 years being: 1.0 per cent, 1.4 per cent, 4.1 per cent, 5.7 per cent, 13.0 per cent, 21.6 per cent and 32.2 per cent respectively. In subjects aged under 75 years, the prevalence of dementia was slightly higher in men than women, and consistent with other findings (Prince 1985); for those aged 75 years and over the prevalence was higher in women. Significantly as Hofman *et al.* (1991: 736) commented, the prevalence figures 'nearly doubled with every five years of increase in age'. This has obvious implications given that the greatest increase in the ageing population is among those aged 85 plus (Health Education Authority 1998), a point reiterated in the most recent review of mental health services for older people in the UK (Audit Commission 2000).

Such a concomitant age-related rise in the prevalence of dementia has been recognized for some time, and in the UK the Alzheimer's Disease Society (1997: 25) (now the Alzheimer's Society) provided a detailed breakdown on the estimated numbers of people with dementia by British health authority and suggested that, by the year 2021 there will be around 900,000 people in the UK with some form of dementia. To plan appropriately for this, the Alzheimer's Disease Society (1997) urged health authorities to make the assessment of need of people with dementia one of their 'key priorities'. It would also be advisable to include the needs of carers of people with dementia who are more prone than other caregiving groups to experience feelings of depression, burnout and loneliness (for comprehensive literature reviews see Dhooper 1991; Kuhlman *et al.* 1991; Downs 1994; Keady 1996). Despite this the Audit Commission (2000) review identified significant gaps in service provision for people with dementia and their carers, especially in primary health care settings. This has to be a cause for concern given that at least one-third of people with the most severe dementia are still living in the community (Audit Commission 2000).

Depression

Late-life depression should not be considered as a natural part of the ageing process (Salzman 1997) and is associated with reduced life expectancy and quality of life (Bartels *et al.* 1997). In an early survey of 997 older people aged 65 and over living in the community with depression, Blazer (1982) reported the frequency of symptoms as shown in Table 7.1.

Similar findings have been reported in numerous community-based surveys (see for example Glass *et al.* 1997; Livingston *et al.* 1997; Dent *et al.* 1999), with the literature also suggesting that older people, despite experiencing considerable symptoms, are less likely than younger people to take up mental health services (Cuijpers 1998). This is of particular concern as studies indicate that a combination of feelings of helplessness and hopelessness are predictors of suicidal thought or actions in people with depression (for a review see Ashton and Keady 1999), and it is a salient reminder that in the UK the incidence of suicide among older people over 65 is three times that in the 15–24 age group, and that older people are more likely to repeat the attempt than those in other age groups (Department of Health 1997a). Suicide rates are particularly high for males (Murphy 1988; Clarke and Fawcett 1992) with, in 1990, the suicide rate for those aged 65 and over being 50 per cent higher 'than the average for the population as

Table 7.1 Frequency of symptoms in a community sample of older people with depression (per cent)

Emotional	
Worry	28
Loneliness	10
Low self-esteem	18
Uselessness	35
Sadness	27
Loss of interest	13
Cognitive	
Difficulty concentrating	13
Poor memory	21
Pessimism	30
Self-blame	15
Irritability	16
Physical	
Loss of appetite	12
Fatigue	22
Sleep difficulty	26
Restlessness	25
Constipation	30

Source: Blazer 1982: 26

a whole' (see Ashton and Keady 1999: 344) the incidence being highest in those aged 75 plus (Murphy 1988). This statistic highlights both the need for more targeted intervention, and the necessity for further empirical studies exploring the experience of depression from the perspectives of the older person, their carer and wider support network.

Snowdon (1998: 61) suggests that interventions for older people with depression should be multilayered and encompass:

- environmental changes
- lifestyle changes
- changing outlook and attitudes using cognitive-behavioural therapies (CBT) (see also Koder *et al.* (1996) for a comprehensive review of CBT)
- other psychotherapeutic approaches, for example group, marital, family or interpersonal therapy
- antidepressant medication.

Such a diverse range of interventions requires sufficient numbers of appropriately trained practitioners. This is manifestly not the case, with high rates of undiagnosed and untreated depression being found in community and residential settings (Audit Commission 2000). The situation appears to be most fraught in residential environments where as many as 40 per cent of older people may suffer a degree of depression (Audit Commission 2000). Other obvious gaps in both data and services relate to the needs of depressed older people from ethnic minority groups who may receive less support from their families than accepted wisdom would suggest (Audit Commission 2000).

Older people and HIV/AIDS

There is an emerging body of literature about older people and HIV/AIDS (Rickard 1995; Youdell *et al.* 1996; Marshall 1997; Wright *et al.* 1998), but little in the way of epidemiological studies. The work of Wright *et al.* (1998) is of particular relevance as they argue that AIDS has been termed the 'great imitator' of other mental health conditions, for example with AIDS-related dementia often being confused with Alzheimer's disease (see also Jamieson 1999). Therefore despite the limited literature there is clearly a need for greater awareness and recognition of AIDS in the older population by health and social care practitioners.

Alcohol misuse

Peressini and McDonald (1998) argue that the incidence of alcohol misuse in older people varies between 2 per cent and 10 per cent. Interestingly, a longitudinal study in Liverpool, exploring in detail the drinking patterns of 1070 elderly people over a period of three years, revealed that people generally drink less as they get older (Saunders 1989).

In their study Peressini and McDonald (1998) evaluated a training programme on alcoholism and older adults aimed at health and social service practitioners. The authors argue that a lack of 'specific knowledge' about the nature of alcoholism and its effects on older people prevents practitioners from recognizing, identifying and referring such clients to further support services. Peressini and McDonald (1998) assert that alcohol misuse in older age should figure prominently in the education and training of professional caregivers.

Living arrangements

Adams and Wilson (1996) argue that the living arrangements of older people is a neglected area, describing an elderly population with a mixture of mental health problems living inappropriately in either long stay wards of psychiatric hospitals or in homeless person's hostels. The research undertaken by Adams and Wilson (1996) included interviews with 41 older people with mental health needs who had been rehoused, and clearly illustrates the effect, both positive and negative, that good or poor housing can have on the older person's mental health. Indeed, the authors suggest that much of the support required is not of a specialized kind, but could, instead, be provided by mainstream housing staff with minimal additional training.

Ethnic minority elders

People from ethnic minority groups who have mental health needs face formidable barriers to mental health services, for while under-utilization of services is relevant to the older population generally, it is particularly acute among ethnic groups, with up to 80 per cent of older people from ethnic minorities not receiving the mental health services they require (Biegel and Farkas 1997). Biegel and Farkas (1997) suggests three main areas for practice improvement: first, increasing the numbers of bilingual mental health workers; second, addressing cultural barriers created by mental health services; third, increasing professionals' specialized knowledge of cultural diversity. Mirroring this, Espino and Lewis (1998) further argue that 'special problems' are faced by ethnic minority groups who experience dementia, and that such problems include medication usage, institutional barriers and family care issues. The conclusions of the Audit Commission review reinforce the need for urgent attention to the mental health needs of older people from ethnic minority groups (Audit Commission 2000).

The foregoing has provided a brief overview of some of the numerous issues relating to the mental health needs of older people and their carers. The remainder of the chapter provides some pointers as to how current deficits might be addressed, beginning with the need for a coherent policy framework.

Developing an integrated policy and service framework

As noted in other chapters, policy initiatives in general, and those for older people in particular, are often vague and unspecific. This is especially obvious in relation to the provision of mental health services as a brief historical review demonstrates.

Until the late 1960s older people with mental health needs constituted a largely invisible group, cared for as inpatients in county asylums, or in outpatient clinics at the local general hospital, their care being undifferentiated from that of other people with mental illness. However, in 1973, fuelled by dissatisfaction with this situation the 'old age group' of the Royal College of Psychiatrists was formed, working towards the formal recognition of old age psychiatry as a speciality within the NHS. During the 1970s, largely due to the efforts of this group, policies were initiated providing at least one 'psychogeriatric' consultant in each district (Johnson *et al.* 1997). Subsequently service provision for older people with mental health needs was based on a mixed economy of care including: inpatient assessment/treatment units; long stay accommodation/provision; day hospitals; outpatient or community assessment and management. Although this could be considered to have advanced practice, we would question if real progress was achieved and suggest that there is still room for considerable improvement. Indeed the need for change has been recognized for some time (Alzheimer's Disease Society 1995; Department of Health 1995a, 1996, 1997b, c; NHS Confederation and the Sainsbury Centre for Mental Health 1997; Audit Commission 2000) and was raised in the early 1980s in the influential report *The Rising Tide* (Health Advisory Service 1982).

This report outlined the components of a comprehensive mental health service for older people and recommended that:

> the role in providing support, advice and relief at times of special difficulty to families and primary health and social services is an essential ingredient in a successful comprehensive service.
>
> (Health Advisory Service 1982: 17)

This early, overt commitment to carers and people with dementia was later reinforced by the King's Fund Centre (1984) in a project paper detailing the principles of good practice, which challenged service providers and policy makers to address five key principles based on beliefs about personal empowerment for people with dementia. These five principles (King's Fund Centre 1984: 7–8 abridged) called for an acknowledgement that:

1 People with dementia have the same human value as anyone else irrespective of their degree of disability or dependence.
2 People with dementia have the same varied human needs as anyone else.

3 People with dementia have the same rights as other citizens.
4 Every person with dementia is an individual.
5 People with dementia have the right to forms of support which do not exploit family and friends.

Although not labelled as such, the principles of a person-centred approach are clearly evident here. As the 1980s wore on, government concern over the costs of funding the NHS stimulated a major debate over its purpose and priorities. A fundamental review led by Sir Roy Griffiths (see Griffiths 1988) and the publication of two White Papers – *Caring for People* and *Working for Patients* (Department of Health 1989a, b) – which were to form the blueprint of the NHS and Community Care Act (Department of Health 1990) – changed the landscape of dementia care practice and assessment, and that of older people with mental health needs more generally (Ford and Keady 1997). In particular, the separation of 'health' and 'social' care within the NHS and Community Care Act spelt out new challenges and responsibilities for case management, and transferred primary responsibilities for the social care needs of older people to local authorities (Department of Health 1991a, b).

More recently, the Department of Health's (1997b) *Handbook on the Mental Health of Older People* was published to assist health and social service purchasers to develop local strategies to improve services and achieve the 'Health of the Nation' targets. The first edition of the Health Advisory Service 2000 (1999) report on mental health services for older people in inpatient and community settings set out suggestions for service development, and established benchmarks for coordinated services for older people with mental health needs and their carers. Particular attention was given to the needs of carers and support and supervision for staff at all levels of service delivery and organization, providing a framework which potentially addresses the lack of cohesion so long apparent in respect of mental health and older people.

The need for greater cohesion was clearly indicated in the review of mental health services for older people undertaken by the Audit Commission (2000). This examined in detail the way in which mental health services for older people are organized and delivered in twelve locations throughout England and Wales. Although examples of good practice were identified, the overall picture was one of 'patchy and inconsistent' service delivery, with wide variation in quality and quantity. In terms of overall service development the report concluded that there was a need for

- mental health professionals to provide more training and support for GPs and primary care teams
- more flexible home-based services
- health and social services to work more effectively together to pool information about individuals and to ensure better use of shared resources
- commissioners of health and social care should have better information

about the services they provide, who receives them and how well they are working.

Significantly the report identified marked deficiencies in the way that assessment procedures are conducted and the level and type of support received by family carers. One of the major recommendations was that users and carers should be more fully involved in assessments and be better informed about their care. This requires new approaches to professional working and it is to this area that attention is now turned.

Creating a new vision for professional assessment and intervention

This section draws predominantly on studies concerned with older people with dementia, reflecting (as noted earlier) the relative dearth of sound empirical and theoretical work in other areas. This represents a major gap in the literature, and given the epidemiological data considered earlier, this is an area requiring far more work. Notwithstanding such gaps in understanding, our primary concern in conducting the review was to begin to identify an epistemology of practice for the care of older people with mental health needs, to inform important areas such as assessment. Limitations in competence and discrepancies in assessment practice have been identified for some time (Guilmette and Snow 1992), leading some to argue for the standardization of assessment procedures across disciplinary boundaries (Hamid and Silverman 1995; Audit Commission 2000).

Attention to technical elements of assessment alone is unlikely to result in significant improvements unless accompanied by a change in the culture of care, away from a primarily medical approach, and the belief that 'nothing can be done' for those with irremediable conditions (Iliffe 1994; Audit Commission 2000). Important work began in the field of dementia and, from the mid-1980s onward Dr Tom Kitwood and his colleagues at the Bradford Dementia Group conceptualized a new approach to the social understanding of people with dementia (see Kitwood 1988, 1989, 1990a, b; 1992, 1997; Kitwood and Bredin 1992a, b). Kitwood's theory was underpinned by the need to rebalance the 'technical framing' of dementia and complement it with a philosophy that was constructed from 'personhood' and 'person-centred values' (Kitwood 1988). Kitwood and his colleagues cogently argued that, 'dementia' is not the problem, rather it is 'our' (individual, carer, professional, society) inability to accommodate 'their' view of the world. This, Kitwood and Bredin (1992a) suggested, creates a 'them' and 'us' dialectic tension, which is sustained by the devalued status of someone who has 'demented'.

Kitwood and Bredin (1992a: 10) contended that there was 'no coherent theory of the process of care' for people who have dementia, and in order to address this deficit Kitwood (1988) reconceptualized the dementing process along the following lines:

$$SD = P + B + H + NI + SP$$

where SD refers to senile dementia, which is viewed as the product of a complex interaction between the remaining five elements of the equation:

P = personality, which includes coping styles and defences against anxiety

B = biography, and responses to the vicissitudes of later life

H = health status, including the acuity of the senses

NI = neurological impairment, separated into its location, type and intensity

SP = social psychology which constitutes the fabric of everyday life.

Kitwood (1988) suggested that the elements of this equation account for most of the phenomena associated with the range of dementias, while also explaining the unique course of each person's dementia. This theory highlighted the limitations of care environments and approaches to people with dementia (Kitwood 1990b), which, for Kitwood (1990b), conspired to produce a 'malignant social psychology', inhibiting the full expression of people with dementia. Crucial to the emerging theory was the acceptance of the construct of 'personhood' and recognition that this 'malignant social psychology' had 'beared down powerfully' on those with dementia (Kitwood and Bredin 1992a), with Kitwood (1997) identifying a range of behaviours which he believed created and sustained a hostile environment (see Table 7.2).

Driving Kitwood was his hope that if the elements of a 'malignant social psychology' could be identified, challenged and rectified, then care (both from family and professional carers) could be improved and people with dementia would experience a greater sense of personal 'well-being'. To operationalize his approach a process of Dementia Care Mapping (Kitwood 1990b; Kitwood and Bredin 1992b) for use in formal settings was established (see Brooker *et al.* 1998). More contentiously Kitwood and Bredin (1992a) suggested that changes to the social environment could cause a reversal of the dementing process, or 'rementia', thereby actively challenging the prevailing medical stage theory of dementia. Adopting Kitwood's model has notable implications for the caring professions as people with dementia are now seen as active agents, a position requiring significant changes to professional attitude and culture.

Although this work is not without its critics, particularly of its underpinning research methodology (Adams 1996a), and predominant focus on long-term care environments (Cheston and Bender 1999), it has been enormously influential, providing nurses and other health and social care providers with a rationale for developing better care for people with dementia (see Matthew 1996). Therefore despite criticism, Kitwood's work has been remarkably influential and has engendered a new ethos of care

Table 7.2 Main features of 'malignant social psychology'

Treachery	the use of dishonest representation or deception in order to obtain compliance
Disempowerment	doing for a dementia sufferer what he or she can still do, albeit clumsily or slowly
Infantilization	implying that a dementia sufferer has the mentality or capability of a baby or young child
Condemnation	blaming; the attribution of malicious or seditious motives, especially when the dementia sufferer is distressed
Intimidation	the use of threats, commands or physical assault; the abuse of power
Stigmatization	turning a dementia sufferer into an alien, a diseased object, an outcast, especially through verbal labels
Outpacing	the delivery of information or instruction at a rate far beyond what can be processed
Invalidation	the ignoring or discounting of a dementia sufferer's subjective states, especially feelings of distress or bewilderment
Banishment	the removal of a dementia sufferer from the human milieu, either physically or psychologically
Objectification	treating a person like a lump of dead matter, to be measured, pushed around, drained, filled and so on
Ignoring	carrying on (in conversation or action) in the presence of a person as if they were not there
Imposition	forcing a person to do something, overriding desire or denying the possibility of choice on their part
Withholding	refusing to give asked-for attention, or to meet an evident need
Accusation	blaming a person for actions or failures that arise from their lack of ability, or their misunderstanding of the situation
Disruption	intruding suddenly or disturbingly upon a person's action or reflection, crudely breaking their frame of reference
Mockery	making fun of a person's 'strange' actions or remarks; teasing, humiliating, making jokes at their expense
Disparagement	telling a person that they are incompetent, useless, worthless and so on, giving them messages that are damaging to their self-esteem.

Source: Kitwood 1997: 46–7

which recognizes that the medical model, although making an important contribution, has limitations. In focusing on the person with dementia it has not only moved away from an overtly pathological model but also provided a therapeutic rationale for staff, thereby raising the status of a hitherto neglected and devalued area of practice. This, in turn, has led to far greater emphasis being given to the perceptions of people with dementia and their more creative role in the design and delivery of services (see Goldsmith 1996; Keady 1999).

It is also important to remember that other therapeutic approaches are available with reality orientation, reminiscence and life review, validation therapy and snoezelen receiving specific mention by the Audit Commission (2000). A comprehensive review of these approaches is beyond the scope of this chapter but the Audit Commission identifies a range of further reading.

Although the circumstances of people with dementia have received increased attention, the most extensive literature is on the needs of family carers. Once again an in-depth consideration of this literature is not possible here (see Nolan *et al.* 1996a; Keady 1999 for detailed review). The range of difficulties that carers face and the support they need is now reasonably well understood, however, reflected in the greater clarity apparent in recent policies such as the Carers' National Strategy (see Chapter 2).

Unfortunately these new insights appear to have had relatively little impact, with the limitations of current practice with carers in other settings having already been discussed (see Chapters 3, 4 and 5). These were mirrored in the Audit Commission (2000) review on mental health services in older age, which highlighted the limited involvement of older people and carers in the assessment and planning of care, with particular deficiencies apparent in the support received by carers. For example, from the Audit Commission data only half of carers received an adequate explanation of dementia and its likely impact on their lives, and respondents were not informed as to where they could go for help or even what help was available. Similarly, when choosing a nursing home, most carers did not know what to look for in a quality home nor how to go about selecting a home.

The assessment of carers' needs is clearly still deficient and (as has been argued elsewhere in this book) these are best understood within a temporal framework. Many of the studies underpinning such an approach have emerged from the field of dementia.

Lindgren (1993) for example, outlined the concept of a 'caregiving career' building on Corbin and Strauss's (1988) definition of an 'illness trajectory' described as 'the total organisation of work done over the course (of the illness) plus the impact on those involved with the work and its organisation' (Corbin and Strauss 1988, quoted in Lindgren 1993: 214). The caregiving career is the time in a person's life during which the central focus is on caregiving and a number of studies in dementia have adopted this temporal framework. Other areas of mental health need in older age (such as depression, schizophrenia or anxiety disorders) have not been explored so extensively and further empirical work is urgently needed in these areas.

Lindgren (1993) considers the 'career' in terms of three stages – the encounter stage, the enduring stage and the exit stage – and suggests that each stage is determined by the disease trajectory of the person with dementia. For instance, in the encounter stage, carers become aware of the diagnosis and may need to acquire new skills, in the enduring stage they may have to manage extensive care routines, while the exit stage marks the end of the caring due to the person's institutionalization or death. However, this may signal a premature ending, as carers continue to be involved in caring after placement in a home (see Chapter 5).

Wright (1993) explored the interaction between spouses and people with dementia during the illness trajectory with 30 spouses being assessed at baseline and two years later. Wright (1993) suggests that spousal interactions influence outcomes, with continued in-home care being predicted by high levels of positive spousal interactions, high caregiver commitment, good caregiver health and shorter time as a caregiver (for a comprehensive longitudinal study that supports this analysis see also Sällström 1994).

Other attempts at interpreting the experience of dementia can be found in a number of temporal models (see for instance Hirschfield 1981, 1983; Clarke and Watson 1991; Willoughby and Keating 1991; Kobayashi *et al.* 1993; Taraborrelli 1993; Collins *et al.* 1994; Garwick *et al.* 1994; Harvath 1994), although only a few have drawn upon the experience of people with dementia. For instance, Hirschfield (1983) failed to report on the data collected from seven people with dementia and, instead, focused upon generating a temporal model of care from the carers' perspective. Other studies, for example that by Wuest *et al.* (1994), followed a longitudinal model but argued that the trajectory is universally downward with carers inevitably moving towards a state of alienation from the person with dementia.

This rather negative image of family care and the experience of dementia is not inconsistent with accounts of personal growth and satisfaction that feature in other studies (Motenko 1989; Kobayashi *et al.* 1993; Cohen *et al.* 1994; Nolan *et al.* 1996a). For example the grounded theory study by Kobayashi *et al.* (1993) outlined a seven stage model of caring which highlighted the personal growth and evolving expertise enjoyed by family carers throughout the continuum of care. The study also drew attention to the importance of recognizing non-verbal communication within the caregiving relationship, demonstrating that this form of interaction continues even though there may be no meaningful conversation between participants. In contrast to the negative picture portrayed by Wuest *et al.* (1994), Kobayashi *et al.* (1993) suggested that after working through a period of uncertainty, carers developed feelings of empathy and understanding for the person with dementia. Thus, carers learn to appreciate aspects of the person with dementia and to find other methods of communication.

Building on these earlier studies, and particularly the work of Wilson (1989a, b), Keady (1999) conducted a study which charted the experience of caring for someone with dementia over time, and uniquely, draws on data from people with dementia and integrates these with the accounts of carers. Although exploratory and based on the experiences of small numbers of people (ten) with dementia, this study raises a number of significant issues. In particular it illustrates that people with dementia and their carers frequently work hard at the caring relationship, but often in opposite directions. For instance in the early stages of dementia, the person with memory problems develops ingenious strategies to 'hide' their failing ability, expending considerable time and energy. Eventually the family member begins to suspect that something is wrong and also puts considerable effort in trying to 'discover' what is happening. This situation can continue for some time and sustains a pretence that is generally not productive and may even be destructive, potentially spoiling relationships. One of Keady's (1999) conclusions is that early diagnosis, assessment and support would do much to help resolve potential difficulties by harnessing the positive energy of the person with dementia and their carer to plan a joint approach for the future.

Unfortunately there are often particular difficulties in the early stage of dementia, with general practitioners (GPs) generally lacking the skills and training to support early diagnosis. Exacerbating matters many practitioners see no point in the early diagnosis of what they consider an untreatable condition (Audit Commission 2000). Such a negative view has to be challenged if people with dementia and their carers are to experience an optimum quality of life, and the conduct and standard of assessments of older people and their carers is to improve (Worth 1998; Audit Commission 2000). Despite the crucial role of assessment in community care, a number of issues remain problematic, including: the purpose and process of assessment; comprehensiveness of assessment; joint working in relation to assessment; user empowerment; relating needs to resources; and differences between nursing and social work assessment.

Recent studies have made recommendations about what should be included in the assessment of informal carers, which are summarized in Table 7.3. However, most of these reflect a research rather than a practice agenda and models are needed which facilitate the transition of theoretical ideas into practice.

An attempt has been made by Nolan *et al.* (1998b) who, based on over ten years' research in the field of family care, produced an assessment framework, together with supporting indices that can be used to provide more structure and logic to the assessment of carers' needs. Complementing this there are emerging models which also focus more specifically on the mental health needs of older people, for example the Index of Managing Memory Loss (IMMEL: Keady and Nolan 1996). Further work is needed to identify how such ideas can influence and inform practice.

More generally the literature review also highlights the increased attention being given to the construct of quality of life among older people (Bowling 1998) and its measurement for those with mental health needs (DeLetter *et al.* 1995; Nilsson *et al.* 1996; Stedman 1996; Wills and Leff 1996; Albert *et al.* 1997). Consistent with the conclusions of Chapter 1, it is clear that subjective assessments are more influential in determining happiness, well-being and life satisfaction than are the

Table 7.3 Some key points from the literature review

Effects of caregiving on health and well-being	Burgener 1994; Collins *et al.* 1994; Gallagher and Mechanic 1996; Buffman and Brod 1998
Stress of caregiving	Stevenson 1990; Donaldson *et al.* 1998; Pot and Deeg 1998
Coping and adaptation	Dodds 1994; Kramer 1994; Kramer and Vitaliano 1994; Matsuda 1994
Changing relationships	Spaid and Barusch 1994; Wuest *et al.* 1994
Assessment	Carers (Recognition and Services) Act DoH 1995; Nolan and Caldock 1996; Worth 1998
Assessment tools	Spaid and Barusch 1994; Nolan *et al.* 1995b; Keady and Nolan 1996
Interventions with carers	Corcoran and Gitlin 1992; Davis 1996; Brodaty and Gresham 1997; Heller and Roccoforte 1997; Jansson *et al.* 1998; Wright and Bennet 1998
Gender	Fitting *et al.* 1986; Arber and Gilbert 1989; Harris 1993
Ethnicity	Gonzales *et al.* 1995; Nkongo and Archbold 1995; Guarnaccia and Parra 1996; Connel and Gibson 1997

objective circumstances of the person's life (see in particular Stedman 1996). This has important implications, as following the recent availability of drug treatments in the early stages of dementia, informed debate about determining the impact of such treatments on quality of life is essential (Whitehouse *et al.* 1997). Such ethical and practice dilemmas highlight the need to reconfigure professional practice, education and training.

Reconfiguring professional training and role identity

Notwithstanding some encouraging advances, policy and professional responses to older people with mental health problems and their carers remain largely fragmented and poorly developed across the UK (Audit Commission 2000). This situation is exacerbated by the fact that working with older people with mental health needs has rarely been promoted positively (Jones and Miesen 1992): indeed working with older people with dementia has long been perceived as a negative career choice for health care students (Åström 1986). Furthermore, staff often lack opportunities for clinical supervision and specialized educational development (Department of Health 1994), although recent literature suggests some improvement in this regard (Devine and Baxter 1995; Brocklehurst 1997; Graham 1999).

Despite this, remedial work is needed in a number of areas, especially to improve attitudes towards working with older people with mental health needs and to counter the belief that a deterioration in cognitive functioning rather like isolation, loneliness and depression is a normal part of the ageing process (Social Services Inspectorate 1997). This will mean refocusing attention away from acute care needs and promoting work with older people as skilled and valued. Some indications on a way forward for example have been provided by Adams (1989, 1991, 1994, 1996b, c), who has written extensively about the work of the community psychiatric nurse (CPN) with older people with dementia exploring the application of theoretical models for carers and older people with mental health needs. Adams (1998) suggested that there are three main theoretical approaches to dementia care which he described as care for the carer, the biomedical approach and the psychosocial approach. Adams (1998) argues that none of these models provides a complete account of dementia and the situation of carers, believing that the 'care for the carer' approach neglects the person with dementia, while the other two neglect the family and socio-political context of dementia care (Adams 1998: 615–16). To counter this, Adams (1998) suggests that practice should be based on the notion of listening to the narratives of both the person with dementia and their informal carer, without prioritizing either, a position he describes as follows:

> Nurses need to be more fully aware of the family politics of dementia care within which the interests of each party compete within one another and are voiced in the form of accounts that they give to various people including the mental health nurse.
>
> (Adams 1998: 619)

However, to make this a reality, attention must be given to developing and extending training and educational opportunities so that work with older people with mental health needs is valued by nurses and other professionals.

For example nurses working with older people with mental health problems experience role confusion. Nolan *et al.* (1999a) conducted a focus group involving 50 first level nurses all directly involved in mental health care provision (although not all worked with older people). These authors found that tensions existed between the reality of 'front-line' staff and the policy rhetoric, and that rivalry between mental health professions is still 'rife' (Nolan *et al.* 1999a: 53). Nurses described feeling 'disempowered' and experienced a lack of continuity in the care for people with mental health needs. The authors also found that nursing had split into 'factions', each with poor understanding of the other's role, compounded by the power struggle between the specialist roles of psychiatrists and psychologists. For example the heightened emphasis on psychological therapies, such as CBT and family therapy, meant that nurses no longer saw themselves as 'key players' in the field. Such limited preparation for practice and 'role searching' is definitely indicative of a profession where confidence is low and skills are poorly defined.

Building on this work Nolan *et al.* (1999a) outlined a framework for future practice development in mental health nursing care:

- initial training should place less emphasis on general nursing and hospital based care
- better preparation for assessment of mental health clients, especially risk assessment
- access to good quality clinical supervision
- sabbaticals so that nurses from one discipline can spend time in other areas of nursing.

(Based on Nolan *et al.* 1999a: 53–4)

There is a need for similar work specific to the mental health care of older people, to identify the skills and knowledge required, particularly in terms of assessment. Risk assessment for older people, especially those with mental health needs who live alone, provides a case in point with a paucity of research and policy in this area. One of the few studies in the field of dementia care suggested that in the UK there are 154,000 people living on their own with dementia, with half this total being aged 85 years or over and exposed to increased risk, such as undetected self-neglect, financial exploitation and falls (Alzheimer's Disease Society 1994). Reinforcing the need for practice development, a report by the Department of Health (1997c: 38) outlined the components of a risk assessment as being

- self-neglect
- exploitation
- wandering
- abuse
- injury
- isolation
- financial loss
- damage to property
- risk to others.

This report also suggested that professionals, particularly care managers, had little understanding of mental health 'conditions' and that there is an urgent need for approved practice in this area.

As so little is known about the experience of mental illness in old age, particularly for those who live alone, additional insights are necessary before the policy rhetoric can be turned into practice reality. Furthermore, recent moves towards primary care assessment mean that other practitioners, such as health visitors and practice nurses, have increased opportunity to play a lead role in assessment (Audit Commission 2000). Unfortunately, the literature suggests that practice nurses, for example, do not feel comfortable in such a role (Nolan *et al.* 1999b) and require further support and education (Ford *et al.* 1997; Secker *et al.* 1999). This situation needs to be addressed if the quality of life of people with mental health needs and their carers is not to diminish further.

Conclusion

As this review has highlighted, there remains a great deal to be done if services for older people with mental health problems are to improve. There have also been some important recent developments with, for instance, the Mental Health Foundation (1995) financing a stream of research in the area and the Alzheimer's Society placing an emphasis on quality of life and promoting a research strategy that involves people with dementia and their carers in decision making about grant allocation. Such moves are reflective of a growing empowerment model and are, of course, to be welcomed. However, they need to be accompanied by a reorientation of practice and closer alignment between various professions and agencies.

The arguments that Barker *et al.* (1998) advanced in respect of mental health nursing need to be applied more widely. These authors believe that psychiatric nursing must find its 'proper focus' which by assent means acknowledging people as human beings first and patients with problems second. Such a philosophy mirrors the person-centred approach which has figured so prominently throughout this book. There is an obvious consensus on the appropriateness and relevance of such a model but far less as to how it might be achieved. Work in the field of mental health in older age has provided some important insights most notably in the writings of Kitwood and colleagues. These, together with the themes from other chapters, will be brought together in the final chapter.

8

Older people with learning disabilities: health, community inclusion and family caregiving

Gordon Grant

Elderly people with learning disabilities are a phenomenon of the late twentieth century. Not so long ago short life expectancy prevented the vast majority from experiencing the joys and tribulations of old age. Those few surviving to old age were typically locked away in remote long-stay hospitals or supported by their families, in both cases largely invisible to the outside world. Due largely to improvements in pharmacology and the standard of living and health care since the Second World War, this picture has changed appreciably. Survival to old age is now within the bounds of normal expectations for growing numbers of people with learning disabilities around the world (Hogg and Lambe 1998; Janicki *et al.* 1999).

Precisely because older people with learning disabilities and their families are still emerging in numbers and in voice, the literature about their status in society, their health and their everyday lives is not yet well developed (International Association for the Scientific Study of Intellectual Disabilities (IASSID) and Inclusion International 2000). There is much description but there are many gaps in the theoretical literature and in first-hand accounts from severely disabled older people with learning disabilities themselves. Much of what is written about them is inferred from people with learning disabilities in general. This review seeks to avoid a reliance on this 'generic' literature as far as possible.

Caveats aside, this chapter begins by reviewing evidence about the changing demographics, health status and survival of older people with learning disabilities. It draws upon the emergent literature to highlight how ageing and old age is experienced by this group, reviews the circumstances and roles of older family carers in supporting them and considers strategies for intervention. The chapter ends with some challenges for future service development.

A note on definition

The definition of 'old age' in people with learning disabilities is problematic in age-related and functional terms. There are several reasons. First, some subgroups appear to age much more quickly than others. Age-related changes in the health and functioning of people with Down syndrome for example can be identified during middle age. This has led to an unprecedented increase in research activity connected to ageing, co-morbidity and the life course. Many studies have therefore taken the mid-fifties as a criterion for old age in order to include subgroups who age prematurely, or to observe changes in functional status and expectations for change in normal age-related activities. Finally, for adults with learning disabilities who continue to live in the family home parental support is the norm. This has given rise to an interest in the circumstances and challenges facing elderly family carers, many in their seventies, eighties and nineties, who are still supporting 'pre-retirement' and older offspring.

The definitional diversity of old age in the learning disability literature is accordingly difficult to account for in any attempt at synthesis. For pragmatic reasons, this chapter assumes an age criterion of 60 years for elderly people with learning disabilities and 65 years for family carers since these appear to be becoming the norm in more recent literature. Where other studies are included the age categories will be given.

Most of what we know about elderly people with learning disabilities arises from people who are in contact with or known to health and social care services. This would include most with severe or profound disabilities but exclude those with mild learning disabilities, the majority, who probably live quite well without such services. It is a measure of our present poverty of knowledge that we know very little about survival, health, coping and quality of life among this less severely disabled population in Britain.

Lack of directly comparable population data for developing countries means that wider generalizations about the health and social status of older people with learning disabilities cannot be made at the present time. The World Health Organisation has been called upon to address this very issue through supporting programmes of research in developing as well as developed countries (IASSID and Inclusion International 2000).

Demography

Estimating the growing numbers of older people with learning disabilities poses its own problems, not least those previously mentioned in relation to the age cut-off. For example, using intensive case finding methods Hand's (1994) national survey in New Zealand produced a prevalence of 1.43 per thousand older people aged 51 years and over with wide regional variation. Most surveys have to date concentrated on hospital or service samples of older persons because they are captive groups (see for example Takashida *et al.* 1994; Jones *et al.* 1996; Ashaye *et al.* 1997) to explore subjects as diverse as dimensions of physical and mental health status, neurology and neurochemistry, behaviour and quality of life, but these in effect remain convenience samples with limited generalizability.

Very few studies have used epidemiological or systematically maintained databases and this may lead to sample bias. One exception, a study in Sheffield by Parrott *et al.* (1997), showed that although the proportionate increases in the number of people aged over 80 years over an eight-year period appears to be very high (58 per cent) this adds only a few people each year to the relatively small base number. Prospectively, numbers will also be affected by shifts in fertility ratios so the 'baby boom' generation born in the post-war period will directly result in increased prevalence in the numbers of elderly people with learning disabilities in the coming years.

In the Parrott *et al.* (1997) study a higher prevalence was found on two occasions (2.69 and 2.44 per thousand) though this followed use of one of the country's best maintained local databases about people with learning disabilities. For this reason it is possibly one of the most accurate surveys of the target group anywhere in the world. Other reports have been forced to use estimates of prevalence varying from one to three per thousand because of the methodological difficulties of identifying the target group (Jenkins *et al.* 1993).

Findings about reduced prevalence found in the Sheffield study seem to be borne out by the analysis provided by Rohde *et al.* (1995) of the elderly learning disabled population in the City of Westminster, which also has a very reputable case register. During the period between 1984 and 1994 the number of people aged 61 years and over actually fell from 90 to 77. However the authors suggest that this fall is probably less to do with changes in prevalence and more to do with shifts in fertility patterns in the 1920s and 1930s. Importantly, over the decade the proportion living in community-based residences as opposed to long-stay hospitals had increased dramatically, and there had been a significant rise in the numbers exhibiting challenging behaviours. Reasons for this change in behaviour profile remained subject to speculation but were considered to be associated either with the demands and stresses of community living for individuals or how community norms shape the way others perceive acceptable behaviour. The majority of this population had conditions with no clear aetiology, reflecting the paucity of diagnostic testing in the 1930s and 1940s.

Despite the difficulties in estimating the present and future increases in the number of people with learning disabilities reaching old age, the scale and immediate effects of this contemporary trend are not expected to be so dramatic that they cannot be accommodated by sensible and reasonably well informed local planning.

The effects of ageing

A large number of studies in this field have employed cross-sectional designs and have compared older with younger populations of people with learning disabilities. British longitudinal studies of the health and social status of the older population of people with learning disabilities are virtually non-existent so what we know about the effects of ageing have to be inferred from studies with cross-sectional designs with all their flaws, or from North American and European studies which have deployed longitudinal designs.

Ageing and physical health

Some years ago Moss (1991) speculated that people with learning disabilities aged 50 years or more were a more healthy group than those who die at a younger age due to different mortality, with very many people with profound learning disabilities or multiple physical disabilities dying young. The findings of Cooper's (1998) careful epidemiological study in Leicestershire suggest an alternative view. Comparing people aged 65 years and over with a randomly selected group of younger adults she found that the older group had higher rates of urinary incontinence, immobility, hearing impairments, arthritis, hypertension and cerebrovascular disease. The younger group on the other hand had higher rates of dermatological disorders, congenital heart disease, ear, nose and throat disorders and neurological disorders (excluding Parkinson's disease). The older group was more dependent on drugs for physical illness. Although those with the greatest severity of learning disability are likely to die at a younger age, the effects on physical health of ageing seem from these findings to outweigh the effects of this differential mortality.

Though using a less medically rigorous procedure than Cooper, findings for older people from studies in the United States by Janicki and MacEachron (1984), New Zealand (Hand 1994) and the Netherlands (Haveman *et al.* 1989) are broadly confirmatory in relation to hearing impairments, arthritis, cardiovascular disorders, respiratory conditions and neurological disorders. Cumulative research experience suggests that the target group has rates of common adult and age-related conditions comparable to or higher than that of the general population, but factors relating to specific syndromes (Down, Fragile-X, Prader Willi, for example), associated developmental disabilities (cerebral palsy, epilepsy, for example), lifestyle and environmental factors are considered to play a part in explaining higher rates (Evenhuis *et al.* 2000).

Despite these findings, general practitioners seem to be rather dismissive of the need for regular health checks or hearing and eye tests for people with learning disabilities (Kerr *et al.* 1996), though it is unknown as to whether this reflects lack of interest or lack of knowledge. Whatever the reason for these responses they are reported to create anxieties and distress among older people with learning disabilities and their carers (Grant *et al.* 1995). They demonstrate only too clearly how ignorance or lack of interest from highly trained professionals can compound risks to people's health and well-being.

Participation in diagnostic testing can be quite complicated when older individuals have no one acting in an intermediary capacity as advocates or guardians to represent their interests and concerns. Despite these difficulties comprehensive health assessments appear to be useful in detecting hitherto untreated but treatable medical and dental conditions (Carlsen *et al.* 1994), and specialist assessments, for example of visual acuity, have a vital role in the same respect. However, some conditions like glaucoma can go undetected because testing occurs too late in the life cycle (Evenhuis 1995). In the latter study, specialist assessment was hampered because of fear, refusal, insufficient cooperation or illness in nearly half of the elderly subjects.

Evenhuis *et al.* (2000) have usefully summarized the barriers that can prevent older people with learning disabilities from accessing health care. Although some factors derive from the nature of a person's learning disability or accompanying conditions others are more directly related to the structure and culture of services:

Person-specific
- communication difficulties
- multiple disabilities

Environment-related
- medical history – largely dependent upon staff and carers' observations
- training of staff and carers in assessment, diagnosis and treatment
- education for the patient or client
- informed consent procedures
- time for informant-based medical history-taking
- capacity for dealing with behavioural challenges
- case complexity.

It will be seen that most of the factors mediating access to health services are structural not personal, suggesting that urgent attention be focused on the way in which disabling barriers are created and reproduced within services and society at large (Oliver 1996). A medical deficit or personal tragedy theory of disability which locates thinking within a disability-impairment-handicap framework is clearly an insufficient basis for determining appropriate health and social care intervention and support.

Ageing and mental health

Further work by Cooper (1997a) confirms that, compared to younger adults, older people with learning disabilities are much more likely to have accompanying psychiatric disorders. These are largely accounted for by higher rates of dementia, generalized anxiety disorder and depression. Past history of affective disorder was also present in a larger proportion of the older group. When differences in age ranges are accounted for these findings are broadly in line with those reported by Patel *et al.* (1993). As people with learning disabilities age their need for psychiatric services appears to increase.

Aetiological factors for psychiatric disorders were not examined in Cooper's (1997a) study but were considered most likely to include underlying brain damage, epilepsy, genetic syndromes, family history of mental illness, social and developmental factors, and the additional burdens of physical disabilities. Cooper's commentary on psychological factors contributing to risk for future psychiatric disorders in later life basically suggests that these are rooted in life history, social and economic factors, including:

- effects of shifts in patterns of interdependence with parents during the life cycle
- long-term effects of past care practices reflecting institutionalism and rejection
- service breaks and transitions
- broken relationships with staff during the 'service career'
- stigma
- limited social networks and lack of a close confiding relationship
- low income and relative poverty
- lack of valued roles (paid work, marriage/partnership, parenthood)

These findings are significant in that they suggest the need to rethink the constitutional elements of epidemiological databases for this population.

Thorpe *et al.* (2000) have summarized the situation thus:

> Stressors may be multiple, and include separation from or death of a parent, loneliness and sudden relocation. Unfortunately, little is known about quantifying these influences on age-related changes in persons with intellectual disabilities. However, the general consensus of clinicians in the field is that all perceived symptoms need to be evaluated in a broad context, and not necessarily attributed to one individualized factor but explored as part of a complex interaction of the individual with the environment.
>
> (Thorpe *et al.* 2000: 1)

The authors also suggest that the magnitude of individual adverse reactions to stressors might be accelerated because of cognitive impairment, poor self-esteem and poor perception of self-competence due to repeated adverse life experiences over the lifespan and poor social support (Thorpe *et al.* 2000: 1).

Ageing and dementia

Epidemiological studies suggest that rates of dementia in older people with learning disabilities are around 13 per cent for those aged 50 years and over and 22 per cent for those aged 65 years and over (Moss and Patel 1993; Cooper 1997b), these being about four times higher than one would expect from an age-matched general population (Cooper 1999). Dementia in people with Down syndrome occurs at a substantially higher rate, growing from 2 per cent for the age group 30–9 years, 9.4 per cent for those aged 40–9 years, 36.1 per cent for those aged 50–9 years and 54.5 per cent for those aged 60–9 years (Prasher 1995). Risk factors are still largely uncharted but it is felt that the ease of detection of dementia at the early onset stage in people with Down syndrome may help in the search for an understanding of aetiology, prognosis and ultimately treatment relevant to the general population.

Clinical presentation of symptoms is not always easy to understand for reasons linked to life-history factors discussed earlier, and it is difficult to disentangle symptoms relating to dementia and depression in the target group (Harper and Wadsworth 1990). Furthermore, management can be extremely taxing and complex even when a clear diagnosis has been made. For example, Tony, his sister and brother-in-law were visited by the author as part of a study on family care and provide a good illustration:

> Tony had lived at home with his parents until they died when he was in his thirties. When I first visited Tony he had moved in with his sister, Frances, and her husband, Geoff. He was now aged 51 years. Tony had Down syndrome but during his forties his behaviour started to change. His former ebullient and expressive personality gave way over a period of years to one which was withdrawn and uncooperative. Tony appeared to lose social skills he had formerly gained. Frances and Geoff initially put this down to Tony's sense of loss following his parents' death. Some years later, and much to his sister and brother-in-law's embarrassment, he would forget to button his trousers and attempt to put his jacket on upside down. In addition he occasionally had falls, incurring serious cuts and bruises which required trips to the local hospital A&E department. As a result Frances and Geoff became increasingly protective towards Tony and kept him away from specialist services, though part of this was due to their feeling that they might be accused of maltreatment were they to report Tony's vulnerability to accidents to the local community learning disability team. Tony's increasingly uncooperative behaviour goaded his brother-in-law into anger and quite frequent verbal abuse, reinforcing even further the tactics of withdrawal from services by Frances and Tony. Matters reached a potential breaking point when Frances became overwhelmed by the constant personal care, Tony's night-time wandering, his long silences, and her husband's refusal to help. Tony was subsequently admitted into nursing

home care after efforts at putting a home support package in place failed.

The lived realities of dementia among older people with learning disabilities are largely uncharted but would appear to present major challenges for researchers and others keen to understand how people make sense of major cognitive and accompanying behavioural and physical changes in their lives.

The experience of ageing

The work of Robert Edgerton and his colleagues in the United States has a special significance in shedding light on the lived experience of people with learning disabilities (for example Edgerton 1967; Edgerton *et al.* 1984; Edgerton and Gaston 1991). Spanning the decades, and using longitudinal participant observation methods, ethnographic data have been collected from and about people with mild learning disabilities who live independently in order to understand how they manage and adapt in potentially hostile community environments. More recent work from this team has concentrated on survivors who are now elderly. Additional research has been carried out in relation to elderly learning disabled people living either in family or community residential homes.

Edgerton *et al.* (1994) report that there is considerable diversity in health status and access to health care among both samples. Despite this there were some very important commonalities. Very few people made any attempt to exercise on a regular basis, even when it had been recommended as part of a rehabilitative programme. Only one person consistently avoided a high fat, high sugar diet. Many were overweight. Though there was little evidence of drug or alcohol dependency, many smoked cigarettes heavily despite the advice of relatives and care providers. Few had understanding of the relationship between smoking, diet, exercise and health. Very few were able to offer even basic information about their ailments or worries. Doctors were often found to rely on informed guesswork about appropriate medications and were unaware about drug hoarding evident among some individuals. People living in regulated residential settings on the whole had their health care needs regularly monitored, though infantilizing care practices by staff sometimes led to errors of diagnosis by doctors. In contrast, drug hoarding and its attendant risks were more in evidence among those people living by themselves. All had difficulty determining when they were in need of health care, communicating their needs to others, and understanding how to cooperate in treatment plans.

The communication problems among this older group of people heightened the risks of doctors overlooking necessary medical and surgical procedures, with a number of serious cases coming to light. Gender specific procedures like mammograms, cervical smears or prostate examinations were overlooked. It was surmised that this might be because people tend to think of people with learning disabilities as asexual or that they are equated with groups of low income minority elderly patients among whom such poor practices have been described (Yeatts *et al.* 1992).

Studies have shown that older people with learning disabilities who have verbal skills do display insights into age-related changes in their personal and social lives. Some years ago, Erickson *et al.* (1989) showed that individuals had very varied perceptions about growing older. In this sample of individuals (mean age 62 years) some wished to dissociate themselves from the ageing process while others had more concrete concerns about ageing, ranging from issues about sedentary lifestyles, changes in employment status, loss of mobility and reduced social contacts, fears about incipient ill-health, and recognition that ageing ultimately heralds death. Some were more optimistic about their future lives than others, especially in relation to their use of leisure time. Individual planning or person-centred planning systems would need to be more widely available (Felce *et al.* 1998) for such aspirations and concerns to be picked up and acted upon however.

A growing body of British literature has in recent years begun to explore the everyday life experiences of older people with learning disabilities in a range of living environments (Grant *et al.* 1995; Walker and Walker 1996; Fitzgerald 1998, Walker and Walker 1998). What emerges is a picture of a group, or rather groups, of people who are in many ways living on the fringes of society. They are in the community but not of it in so many ways: their personal finances are often controlled by others; those living 'independently' are highly dependent upon the welfare state, and live in relative poverty not only because their incomes are low but also because their concept of monetary values lands them in financial trouble; difficulties are reported in forming and in maintaining personal relationships based on intimacy, affect and reciprocity – often because people are 'retired' from day services or rehoused away from friends, and sometimes because friends move away or die; the sense of loss following bereavement or from lost contact with family, friends and key others can be profound and kept concealed; the difficulties of gaining admission to and acceptance by generic facilities like 'integrated' clubs and societies remind them that their 'differentness' is somehow more than superficial; and occasional taunts from neighbours and young people about their demeanour or dress code can remind them that their citizenship status is yet to be fully accepted by others even if it is rightfully claimed.

Using the life-history method, Todis (1992) has carefully described how social support can be perceived very differently by two older people with learning disabilities and how their perceptions affect the way in which their support is negotiated:

The two respondents, Wilbur (70 years) and Grace (60 years), first met at a sheltered workshop and married ten years ago. They lived in their own apartment. Mutually supportive of one another, Wilbur and Grace had a greatly expanded social network following their marriage. However, their new life together also obviated the need for family members to visit quite so frequently. Lying at the heart of Wilbur's stance in relation to support that is offered from services is whether it is perceived as help or as an attempt to control his and Grace's lives. The acceptability of help appeared to be contingent upon an appreciation of life's minutiae – in Wilbur's case this was tied to different dimensions of his identity, most notably his disability identity, to his self-perceived competence and to his own constructs of what might or might not make him eligible for services. For Grace, different factors were evident. Her stance was one predicated on support being unconditional. She wanted people in her support network to value her for who she was and not for what she might be, even if this might make other people's lives easier. Indeed she was reported to fear becoming more self-sufficient precisely because she would make it easier for her family to be free not to care for her any more.

What this case illustration captures is that in old age people's identities and self-concept continue to be shaped by the way society as a whole reproduces disability and ageism. This particular group of people do appear to suffer a double jeopardy in this connection (Walker and Walker 1996) – their chronological age separates them at an arbitrary point from former associates and possibly also from specialist learning disability services, while their learning disability continues to bar them from many local social institutions – and as a result their struggles to lead a community included life can be multiplied.

Surprisingly little has been written about gender issues in later life among people with learning disabilities though women's health and related issues were the subject of a report recently submitted to the World Health Organisation (Walsh *et al.* 2000). This report basically suggests that such fundamentals as women's sexual health through the life course and in later life, healthy living, public health related to women's needs and concerns, and women's own social constructions of health all require urgent investigation and action at an international level.

Residential options

There are no national statistics relating to residential provision for older people with learning disabilities in the UK. Local surveys show, however, that individuals are dispersed among a variety of residential services and community living options. The detailed survey conducted by Hogg and Moss (1993) of people with learning disabilities aged 50 years and over showed that 14 per cent were living at home with families, 24 per cent were in long-stay hospitals, 21 per cent in group homes and other forms of supported accommodation, 35 per cent were in hostels and 6 per cent were in sheltered housing of some kind. Hospital closure and resettlement will have a major impact on such figures in the next few years.

In their review report Hogg and Lambe (1998) note that there has been a dearth of research about how these different living arrangements impinge on people's lives. In the absence of clear national policy for this group of older people it would have to be concluded that where they live, how they live and the quality of their lives is very largely adventitious. As these authors point out we do not know whether older people with learning disabilities, especially those with milder learning disabilities who are adept at 'passing' (Edgerton 1967) or 'making out' in the community, figure among the homeless population. Neither do we know what numbers may be detained in secure accommodation or in prison.

The analysis provided by van Gennep (1995) of older people (mean age 65 years) in Dutch institutions and community homes showed that over a five-year period there were some biologically conditioned decreases in functioning relative to sensory-motor functions, continence, physical and mental health, but adaptive behaviour did not decrease as long as the quality of care was good. What seemed to make the difference was what he termed a 'development-orientated' attitude among staff towards their role and function.

A subsequent study by Jones *et al.* (1996) of older people (mean age 62 years) in UK staffed community-based homes drew some similar conclusions. Interestingly, age was found to be related to better quality of life in relation to decision making and community inclusion, both of which reflect a commitment to a person-centred service. Age was found to be associated with greater self-help skills, suggesting that such skills may in some respects mediate the opportunity to make choices and control one's life. The earlier study by McGuire *et al.* (1991) of older residents in two community homes (mean ages of residents 74 years and 68 years respectively) also showed people adapting positively in their new home environments after many years of institutionalization. Neither home reported consistent disruptive or maladaptive behaviours in residents despite the fact that some had presented 'problem' behaviours like 'voluntary' incontinence and attention-seeking behaviour upon first arrival.

Experience in the United States also clearly demonstrates that where older people with learning disabilities reside, or more particularly what type of residence they live in, can have a major impact on important quality of life domains. It has been shown for example that social inclusion depends less on Activities of Daily Living skills and more on care practices and opportunity structures for forming and maintaining relationships with people inside and outside the domicile (Anderson 1993). Also demonstrated was evidence of inappropriate placements with many individuals living in environments with routines and controls poorly matched to their capacities. These were more characteristic of institutions and large private facilities. In an earlier study Anderson (1989) had drawn some similar conclusions:

> The smaller, community-based residential options such as foster care and small group homes offer considerable advantages, including greater potential integration with the community and more normal living conditions than other settings, together with moderate costs and value orientations that emphasise habilitative rather than medical definition and solutions.
>
> (Anderson 1989: 239)

O'Brien's (1994) commentary on support for people with learning disabilities in their own homes is instructive here. He argues that continued residence remains largely based on patronage and compliance with house rules. There is still a long way to go before it can be claimed that these older people experience a sense of place, control their home and the support necessary to live there, and hold the valued role of tenant or home owner.

Older family carers

Demography

Although (as reported earlier) most elderly people with learning disabilities live in some sort of residential care environment, a minority are still supported in the family home. McGrother *et al.* (1996) found that family caregivers aged 60 and over were responsible for looking after 44 per cent of all adults with learning disabilities who were living in a family home. Hogg and Lambe (1998) estimate that there are between 30,000 and 35,000 caregivers in the UK 60 years of age or older supporting relatives with learning disabilities at home.

For these families there are some good demographic reasons for being concerned about expectations for continued support from this source (Seltzer *et al.* 1991):

- increasing life expectancy for people with learning disabilities may prolong caregiving among older family carers
- as a consequence more siblings may be obligated to assume caring roles during middle age years
- but shifts in fertility ratios towards smaller family size may in future years reduce the supply of sibling carers
- hence the dependency ratio (proportion of caregivers to recipients) seems likely to become less favourable.

Changes in the structure of families, the emergence of black and ethnic minority elders and the impact of divorce may have significant consequences for patterns of family caregiving which remain largely uncharted.

The impact of value driven policy will also have a bearing here with encouragement being given to families to let their disabled offspring leave home at a more age-appropriate time.

Care and support networks

Useful reviews of the literature on older family caregivers of adults with learning disabilities are provided by Roberto (1993) and Hogg and Lambe (1998). The reviewed evidence supports the view that most caring is carried out by women throughout the life cycle. Caring is often depicted as hierarchically organized – the primary carers in most cases being mothers but there is usually a pecking order in how responsibilities become assigned. Caring is almost universally based on perceived reciprocities – even if these are not so obvious to third parties. Older carers do not seem to receive the same level of assistance from services as younger carers. As they age, interdependencies seem to grow between carers and their adult offspring (McGrath and Grant 1993; Todd *et al.* 1993; Prosser and Moss 1996) but we know next to nothing about how this is experienced by people with learning disabilities themselves.

Even after leaving the family home in mid-life, older people with learning disabilities can still be supported by informal family networks, usually comprising of siblings (Bigby 1997). However, their networks are quite small and dense and in Bigby's words 'the lack of intergenerational members, shared relationships and situation-specific friendships makes their informal networks vulnerable to shrinkage' (1997: 342), from which we can infer that this might leave people at risk.

Relationships between the structural and dynamic properties of support networks, the transmission of (family) care and successful ageing in this population remain to be studied through systematic research. Until this is done it will be difficult to determine how best to reinforce and enrich family caregiving for this group. However, successful systematic experimental evaluation of family-orientated case management in families supporting younger disabled children in the United States (Dunst *et al.* 1993, 1994) has given rise to a set of working principles which could form the basis of replications among older adults and their families. The family support principles adopted by Dunst and colleagues are:

- use of active and reflective listening skills as the basis for understanding the needs and concerns of families
- help for families to identify, clarify and prioritize aspirations as well as needs
- importance of proactive as opposed to reactive helping styles
- help that is compatible with the family's own culture
- help compatible with the family's definition of problems and circumstances

- help leading to the acquisition of competences that promote independence
- help carried out in a spirit of cooperation and partnership for meeting needs and solving problems
- locus of decision making resting with the family as a whole.

Evidence reported by Robinson and Williams (1999) suggests that we are a long way from realizing these principles in practice with many carers finding that aspects of their lives concerning their health, housing, work and ability to continue caring had not even been discussed during assessments following the Carers Act 1995.

Non-normative caregiving

Tobin (1996) describes older parents of people with learning disabilities as 'perpetual parents' as they have not finished and may never complete launching their offspring towards a more independent life. In comparison to the vast majority of parents they find their adult child still living at home and making demands on their parenting and caregiving resources. Their adult children do not accomplish what Laslett (1989) refers to as the Second Age, that is maturity, independence, familial and social responsibility, largely because they are unlikely to have benefited from good employment opportunities, marriage and from having children. Carers meanwhile often seek to conceal their continued parenting from peers and neighbours so as to create the appearance of a 'normal' lifestyle; this they often accomplish by severing social relationships and accomplishing their caregiving within a very privatized world. Concerned about the future of their offspring, perpetual parents are threatened by unfinished business as the life cycle nears its end. They harbour anxieties about the future, their own capacity to continue caring, and what will happen to their offspring when they themselves die (Grant 1990; Prosser 1997). Time, in short, has entrapped them in what might be regarded as 'non-normative' circumstances.

However, Tobin's work shows that through caregiving these older parents maintain intimacy, assertiveness and a sense of control which can be missing from the lives of their age-related peers. Suspended in social time, perpetual parents evidently encounter rewards in spite of the threats about what the future might bring. This seems to be confirmed by studies which show older parents to be healthier, have better morale, and report no more burden or stress than parents in younger families of persons with learning disabilities or of family caregivers of elderly persons (Seltzer and Krauss 1989; McGrath and Grant 1993).

Caregiving compensations

The uplifts of caregiving appear to be quite pervasive and occur at all points across the lifespan (Heller and Factor 1993; Beresford 1994; Grant *et al.* 1998) so it would be wrong to presume that they have a unique association with non-normative caregiving.

We know little at present about the latent and manifest dimensions of caregiving uplifts and, as Folkman (1997) has suggested, we need to know much more about the processes that trigger a search for positive psychological states, and the intensity and duration of such states necessary to sustain individuals in their everyday caring. Older family carers represent one group for whom exploring these connections would be very worthwhile.

Planning for the future

The 'unfinished business' described by Tobin (1996) conceals many anxieties older family carers hold about the future. Prosser (1997) reported that in a study of family carers of older adults, only 28 per cent had made any residential care plans. In most cases these carers were committed to maintaining long-term care for their relative for as long as possible. More prevalent were financial plans (63 per cent) but in less than half of these cases guidance from solicitors had been sought, which questions just how legally robust these financial arrangements were. Earlier Grant (1989) had found that over half the family carers in his North Wales study had had a major change of mind over a fairly short period (two years) about the preferred long-term care arrangements for their relative. Such vacillation appears to be quite common.

Many factors are influential when future care arrangements come under consideration (Grant 1990; Heller and Factor 1993; Prosser 1997): changes in family support networks can lead carers to revise their plans; they may find themselves contemplating whether caring will become easier or more difficult; they continue to compare the standards of care they know they can provide against that which they presume of statutory and other services; lack of information about different service options can lead to uncertainties about what is best; some carers prefer to rely on their own resources or wish to seek dependency on the state; other carers adopt a 'bury the head in the sand' approach and avoid discussing options with others because of the pain associated with doing so; and there seems to be a constant 'cost-benefit' calculus where carers review their own needs against those of their family and their disabled relative.

Family carers need much clearer information at an earlier stage in the life cycle about the nature of realistic long-term care options, and about what part they and their relative can play in negotiating an option that meets the 'best interest' criterion. If this is neglected many older carers will struggle on until they reach breaking point when it may be too late to do anything else but deal with the immediate crisis. Heller's (1993) studies for example emphasize that older parents are more likely than younger parents to need help in future planning, in obtaining residential placements, and in finding services.

Coping strategies

In a study of the coping strategies of families of people with learning disabilities, Grant and Whittell (1999) found that compared to their younger peers, older family carers were more resigned to their roles, less dependent on information seeking as a coping strategy, and more accepting of the way things had worked out for themselves. However, they had a well-developed capacity to reframe the meaning of situations which seemed linked to their capacity to draw from personal and religious beliefs more than other carers, possibly reflecting greater religiosity in older people in general. They also showed considerable analytic ability and expertise specific to their situation which younger carers did not always have.

These findings do not support the view that as carers age their resourcefulness declines. The so-called 'wear and tear' hypothesis about ageing does not hold; on the contrary, if anything the adaptation hypothesis is more in evidence. This is important as it suggests that concerns about co-morbidity among the growing numbers of ageing family carers have perhaps been overemphasized, and that resiliency among older family carers has been overlooked just as some believe it has in families in general (Hawley and DeHaan 1996).

However, neither the ingredients nor the precursors of resilience in families are fully substantiated and the capacity of families to 'bounce back' from apparent adversities is far from fully understood (Hawley and DeHaan 1996). The same applies to older family carers. We do know that many of the other coping strategies they describe as useful are held in common with younger family carers (Grant and Whittell 1999): for example having a pool of tested coping strategies from which they can choose; being able to match the appropriate coping strategy to a particular demand; and, as mentioned above, being able to reframe the meaning of some challenges as non-problematic or normative so that they feel easier to deal with. However, we do not know if:

- the loss of external resources for coping (support network members through death or moves, reduction of income, reluctance to use formal services for example) means that older family carers have to depend more on their own internal resources (experience, expertise, dispositions, analytic ability and so on) which they therefore become practised in using, or
- such external threats lead to an over-dependence on support from their disabled relative, or
- caring over the life cycle in itself leads to the steady accumulation of expertise and competence.

As Titterton (1992) has suggested there are disappointingly few analytic typologies of coping styles available which might throw light on the differential nature of reaction. It also remains the case that structural factors linked to differential reaction in coping terms are not well understood among older family carers – the influence of age, gender, socio-economic group, race and ethnic identity being particular examples.

Intervening in people's lives

A wide range of interventions for supporting elderly people with learning disabilities and family carers has been reported in the literature. Many of these accounts are descriptive rather than the product of systematic evaluation research. Links between process and outcome are still therefore rather tenuous in many cases. Good description, nevertheless, is necessary as a first step towards robust evaluation. Emergent practices are considered below.

First, however, a conceptual marker is important. Expounding the virtues of social systems theory to the design of interventions with older people with learning disabilities, Dossa (1990) draws on Bogdan and Taylor's (1989) 'sociology of acceptance'. The basic idea is that people at risk of being marginalized by virtue of both age and learning disability are able to have meaningful relationships with other people. They argue that four factors are crucial in this respect:

- *Attributing thinking to the other* – this is seen as being accomplished through an appreciation of non-verbal communication, sensitivity to intuitive elements and the ability to empathize.
- *Seeing individuality in the other* – this entails viewing people as unique, intact individuals with personal identities which set them apart from other individuals, an appreciation of which requires an understanding of biography, motivations and feelings.
- *Viewing the other as reciprocating* – this involves looking upon individuals as resourceful, socially and materially, and capable of entering into relationships where reciprocities can be found.
- *Defining social place for the other* – this requires a sensitivity to all the possibilities for people to occupy an important place in the everyday lives of other people in their personal and community networks.

Dossa (1990) and Bogdan and Taylor (1989) view these factors as humanizing sentiments central to the formation of relationships and the construction of humanness. As such they are representative of a societal view which values the communal, reciprocal and cooperative, coming as they do as an antidote to the market-exchange perspectives prevalent in the 1980s. Social systems based interventions modelled in the above way would seem to have obvious applications to policies which emphasize community inclusion.

There can be major difficulties in realizing such objectives when individuals exhibit inappropriate behaviour. However, the nursing intervention described by Mooney *et al.* (1995), based on principles of applied humanism, seemed to offer some promise in this connection. Patients, average age 68 years, were residents in a US nursing home. The aim was both to manage inappropriate behaviour and simultaneously assist people in their efforts to develop equitable adult relationships. This was accomplished through avoiding punishment, seeking to ensure success, enabling individual decision making, exposing the logical consequences of decisions, supporting gentle interventions and finally teaching for behaviour change. Monitored over twelve months the incidence of disrobing, public masturbation, sitting on the floor, aggressiveness, grabbing, eating inedibles and pilfering was significantly reduced and sustained.

Cotten and Spirrison (1991) have reported those with mild and moderate learning disabilities as equating retirement with sadness and death. Primary preventive interventions like counselling for individuals who are going to be relocated have been described, but not yet evaluated, as relevant in this connection though it seems that friendship losses and their significance to individuals can easily be overlooked when older people retire from day services (Foelker and Luke 1989; Grant *et al.* 1995).

Research also suggests that simple forms of instrumental enrichment can lead to improvements in the cognitive functioning of people with learning disabilities at different points in the adult life cycle. Lifshitz (1998) has demonstrated for example that for different age groups cognitive functioning can be quite easily improved, provided that relevant stimuli are introduced. The outcomes, though based on rather abstract testing procedures, underline the point that care staff should maintain hopes and aspirations for those in their care, seek to provide them with individualized intellectual challenges, and exploit varied forms of instrumental enrichment afforded by care environments.

Faux and Seideman (1996) have shown that there is still a long way to go in supporting families with children and adults with learning disabilities. The 72 parents in their sample felt that many health care professionals failed to respect themselves and their relatives, ignored their expertise in managing affairs and rarely listened to them. By contrast four factors were highly valued by families in their interactions with health professionals: the view that the family unit is unique, resourceful and expert; recognition of the family's definition of what constitutes the 'good life'; a preparedness to relinquish stereotyping families in an effort to exploit partnership working; and the favouring of facilitative interventions based on an empathy with family concerns and a preparedness by professionals to operate in an open and accountable manner.

Life review systems based on an analysis of family ecology (Kropf and Greene 1993) and work aimed at enabling families to assume case management roles (Seltzer 1992) appear to be empowering techniques which are capable of enabling people to take control of their lives and reduce dependency on services.

Finally Racino and Heumann (1992) argue that political processes which involve building coalitions between older people with learning disabilities and other interest groups should constitute part of an agenda for action. To this end they suggest four steps: develop and maintain a sense of personal empowerment; form political coalitions with other interest groups; devise strategies to increase networking between interest groups; and lastly debunk the myths of ageing and disability through self-examination and media campaigns.

Nurses and other health care professionals have a responsibility to draw from these direct and indirect methods of intervention, including those focusing on the individual, the family or communities of interest in support of elderly people with learning disabilities and family carers. However, it is not yet clear whether there is consensus on these points, nor for that matter whether they are best carried out by nurses or shared between those professional groups constituting multidisciplinary and other teams. This in turn raises important questions about service models and planning arrangements.

A confusion of values and models?

At the moment there appear to be three competing models for the planning and design of services for this population:

- the 'age-integrated' model in which a cradle to grave commitment is given in the form of a learning disability dedicated service
- a 'specialist' model in which older people with learning disabilities are provided with services dedicated to their needs
- a 'generic' model in which services are shared with elderly people and the wider population at large.

At the moment opinion seems to favour a generic model backed up by specialist services dedicated to people's needs on the basis that this would most likely strengthen the commitment to community inclusion and emancipation (Hogg *et al.* 2000). However, expert opinion expressed in this same report also stresses the need for further research into this question:

> research is called for into . . . the conditions under which the health and social needs of older people with intellectual disabilities can be met within the context of generic services, and the extent to which additional specialist provision is required.
>
> (Hogg *et al.* 2000: 14)

Unfortunately, there is little concerted or coordinated action on this issue in the UK at this time. Policy thinking seems largely to have ignored and marginalized this potentially vulnerable group. For example, the detailed good practice guide published by the NHS Executive (1998) about the commissioning and provision of health services for people with learning disabilities contains virtually no reference to older people and no guidance specific to their unique circumstances. Confirming this neglect, an analysis of community care plans in the UK showed that most made no specific reference to older people with learning disabilities and in the accompanying national survey of social services departments, NHS trusts and directly managed units 82 per cent indicated that there was no policy in relation to this group, with 74 per cent indicating an absence of specific staff training (Robertson *et al.* 1996). Of course it is possible to argue that there is no need for a policy about older people with learning disabilities on the grounds that they should be treated in the same way as other people with learning disabilities or with other elderly people. Evidence based on people's personal experiences cited earlier suggests that there are likely to be dangers in leaving matters to the application of broad principles since these overlook the specific and differentiated needs of this group.

Rooted in the principle of normalization, the five service accomplishments outlined by O'Brien and O'Brien (1991) have had a major influence on the design of learning disability services both in the UK and in many other countries. They emphasize community presence, participation, choice, respect and competence. This value standpoint has worked very well in reorienting thinking in a human rights direction and towards community inclusion. However, there have emerged rather different conceptualizations of quality outcomes for individuals with disabilities. Felce and Perry (1996) for example suggest a schema which uses both objective and subjective assessments of life conditions and personal satisfaction with regard to physical, material, social and emotional well-being, development and activity; Bach and Rioux (1996) advocate a social well-being approach which is seen as conditioned by self-determination, equality and democratization; while Renwick and Brown (1996) adopt an opportunity-constraint model in which quality of life is constituted in terms of being, belonging and becoming (see also Chapter 1 this volume). All of these models are yet to be tested against the circumstances, however, and more particularly the lived experiences of older people with learning disabilities themselves.

However, each of these approaches suggests the importance of individual and environmental factors, and the links between them, in people's lives which shape health and quality of life outcomes. This would in turn suggest the need for a closer appreciation of

- the perceived dimensions of an individual's personal and public identities
- materialist and metaphysical dimensions of an individual's self concept
- inner and external resources from which individuals can draw in making sense of the world around them
- the relationship between where people are (the present) and where they wish to be (the future)
- the older person's own social constructions of what helps.

Robust theoretical frameworks are also required for purposes of evaluating how services can best support older people with learning disabilities and their family carers. Family and social systems models (Dunst *et al.* 1993, 1994) which have been applied to interventions with disabled children and families appear to offer great potential here in that they have demonstrated the associations between outcomes at the level of the individual, the carer and the family as a whole. Older people with learning disabilities deserve the same attention to their needs but this will mean placing them higher up the priority list for research and service development. The first requirement would appear to be the development of a national service framework which recognizes the needs and aspirations of this group.

9

Integrating perspectives

Mike Nolan, Sue Davies and Gordon Grant

health professions and policy makers more generally are recognising that effective interventions require a dialogue between the abstract knowledge of professionals and the particular, situated knowledge of those who use services or are on the receiving end of policy interventions.

(Barnes 1999: 15)

An understanding of illness that reunites the psychological with the experiential will, it has been suggested, require a far richer and more varied conception of evidence than that previously at stake in 'evidence-based' medicine, taking more seriously patients' conceptions of their own values and goals.

(Evans 1999: 19)

autonomy as an isolated value is incapable of underpinning any shared, societal responsibility for the health of all its members, including the least advantaged. As health inequalities widen (both within and between societies) the moral claims of alternative communitarian values become more urgent.

(Evans 1999: 24)

The dawn of a new millennium provides an almost irresistible opportunity to reflect upon the past and to anticipate the future and commentators in the fields of health and social care have not proved immune to temptation. Dargie *et al.* (1999), for example, in summarizing the results of a major exercise on policy futures within the health service conducted under the auspices of the Nuffield Trust identify a number of trends and consider their potential implications for the delivery of health care until 2015. Particularly relevant in the present context is the need to articulate more clearly the rights and expectations of older people within an integrated policy and planning framework in which an increasingly sophisticated and well-informed public have ever rising expectations with regard to both the length and quality of their life. They argue that an adequate response will require an agenda for health based on new, innovative and long-term strategic planning which reorientates policy towards individual experience and, in relation to older people, calls for the development of broader and more holistic quality of life indicators embedded within a service delivery system which places a proper valuation on care.

The need for a fully integrated policy framework is also unequivocally promoted in the field of social care and welfare to address the 'substantial and persistent' inequalities that older people experience (Bernard and Phillips 2000). In advancing their arguments Bernard and Phillips (2000) note that for too long, social policy for older people has been bedevilled by piecemeal and ad hoc developments. They accordingly call for an explicitly value-based approach relevant for an ageing society as a whole rather than just that section of the population that happens to be aged. They advocate four sets of values which should underpin such an integrated policy:

- a positive, intergenerational life course perspective
- the need to combat all forms of discrimination
- an empowerment model which focuses on citizenship and voice to create new ways of working with older people
- the need for both critical commentary and action.

In many ways such conclusions mirror the contents of the preceding chapters of this book, with the latter point being particularly pertinent. As we noted in the Introduction, one of our primary purposes was to explore critically currently prevalent notions of empowerment, participation and involvement within the context of groups of potentially vulnerable older people and their carers who need support to maintain their quality of life. Although policy considerations are clearly important, and we shall comment on these briefly later, our main emphasis has been on the delivery of direct care in order to identify ways in which more reciprocal and equitable relationships might be promoted and maintained. Our agenda was ambitious, to begin to articulate an epistemology of practice and to rise to the challenge identified by Davies (1998) of bringing competence and caring into a new alliance. We did not intend this simply as an intellectual task, although there is much conceptual work to be done in developing a social theory for better understanding ageing and later life (Harper 2000). We rather hoped that any framework emerging from the literature reviews would have practice relevance and provide a mechanism to unite services in a way which addresses the needs not only of older people and their carers but also of professionals and other paid carers. We believe that the preceding chapters have reinforced the need for a broader, integrative framework. Despite the distinctive and varied needs and circumstances of the interest groups reviewed in Chapters 3 to 8 we identified some important and recurrent themes.

Not surprisingly the literatures reviewed reflected a range of notions such as the promotion of independence, the development of empowerment, participation and involvement and the capturing of 'real experience'. Such concepts constitute the 'new language' of social policy in the 1990s (Bernard and Phillips 2000) and appear to be ubiquitous in the policy arena (Barnes 1999). However, Harper (2000) argues that the shift in emphasis has been rhetorical rather than real, and the conclusions of all the present contributors are largely consistent with such a position. They also highlight the relative absence of a coherent and clearly articulated policy response to the needs of the various constituencies considered.

Encapsulating many of the tensions identified was the pervasive influence of person-centred care, what this might mean, its implications for the design, delivery and evaluation of services and particularly for the relationships between older people and family and formal carers. Central to many of these debates was the importance of understanding subjective meanings and experiences and of recognizing these as constituting legitimate expert knowledge, of a different but equally important type to that held by service providers.

In this concluding chapter we attempt to synthesize themes which emerged throughout the book and to outline a framework which we hope will provide a way toward the development of reciprocal and mutually reinforcing relationships between older people and those providing help and support, from both family and formal services. Consistent with our original aims the main focus will be on the delivery of direct care. It is important first to consider this within the broader policy context.

Towards an integrated policy framework

The tendency for policies for older people to be couched in the language of general principles was noted in the early 1990s (Henwood 1992), the lack of an overall vision still being apparent on both sides of the Atlantic (Easterbrook 1999; Kane 1999). Largely as a consequence services have been fragmented and often lack coherence and direction. Easterbrook (1999) comments tersely that they comprise a 'hotchpotch of innovation and good practice coupled with instances of poor standards, neglect and incompetence'. As Dalley (2000) contends, the vision of seamlessness promoted by successive governments remains as elusive as ever and has proved resistant to repeated exhortations for change. Recent empirical studies bear out such conclusions, with limited evidence of involvement and change for older people and their carers, leaving some with the only option of refusing the services offered (Hardy *et al.* 1999).

If this represents the overall situation of older people generally, it is even starker for certain groups such as those with palliative care needs, mental health problems and learning disabilities. As Chapters 6, 7 and 8 indicated, there has been a dearth of both theoretical and empirical work in all these areas with consequent gaps in our knowledge and understanding. For instance in the field of palliative care it is clear that older people are generally disadvantaged and those with non-cancer conditions virtually ignored. The empirical data collected by Seymour and Hanson vividly illustrate the sense of being abandoned that can be experienced by those in their last year of life. Similarly, dementia aside, Ferguson and Keady (this volume) conclude that the mental health needs of older people have been consistently overlooked. Moreover, even for people with dementia and their carers the recent Audit Commission (2000) report points to poorly developed services, especially in primary care. Possibly the most telling picture is painted by Grant, who concludes that older people with learning difficulties are all but invisible in policy terms, and while they may be in the community they are 'not of it'.

Although perhaps not invisible the needs of older people from ethnic minority groups are similarly poorly understood. While ethnic minority groups were specifically included in the literature search strategy we adopted no coherent or comprehensive account could be located.

The limited attention accorded to all the above groups exacerbates the existing disadvantage they experience, disadvantage which is further heightened by stereotypical and fatalistic attitudes among certain practitioners. For instance, efforts to promote early diagnosis in dementia are often thwarted as such knowledge is seen to provide little advantage in what is perceived as an incurable and progressive condition (Audit Commission 2000). Similarly Grant (this volume) vividly highlights the structural and attitudinal barriers that inhibit access to services such as health promotion for older people with learning disabilities who would clearly benefit from such an approach. Moreover, as Janet Nolan notes in Chapter 4 on community and primary care, such barriers, although perhaps less pronounced, also apply to older people more generally.

Therefore at a time when it is asserted that the government will not tolerate poor care for older people (Hutton 1999), it is clear that disadvantage is not only prevalent, but likely to increase, with evidence suggesting that there is greater distance developing between those who have access to adequate health and social care resources and those who do not (Dargie *et al.* 1999; Evans 1999; Bernard and Phillips 2000).

We contend that even more subtle and pernicious forms of disadvantage and discrimination are also emerging which, if not checked, could disempower substantial numbers of the most vulnerable older people. These relate to the present emphasis placed on the promotion of independence and autonomy as the watchwords of health and social policy (Dalley 2000). The emergence of 'successful ageing' was described in Chapter 1, as were concerns about the potential impact of such a movement for individuals unable to aspire to the criteria of success. Others voice similar concerns. Scheidt *et al.* (1999) for example note that a model of successful ageing based primarily on the absence of disease, high mental and physical functioning and active engagement in life has been widely, if uncritically, accepted and is being used as a blueprint for further research by many sectors of the scientific community and prestigious funding sources. Such values have also been transferred to the public domain resulting in a plethora of 'elixir-like guidelines promoting the new mantra'. While these may make a refreshing change from the 'misery' perspective on ageing (Scheidt *et al.* 1999) the result is likely to be new and invidious forms of 'categorical thinking' based on an increasingly narrow conceptualization of successful ageing which makes a virtue out of being healthy. This has potentially dire consequences for those who are not. Given the diversity of ageing, Scheidt *et al.* (1999) rail against a 'one size fits all approach', promoting instead a model which recognizes the dynamic losses and gains that accompany ageing.

Adopting a similar stance Feldman (1999) forcibly argues for the need to challenge the 'romantic tendencies to valorise the positive aspect of ageing' and urges us to refuse to create a 'new dualism of super ageing in which story-lines of physically fit, creative, active, adventurous ageing become the new unachievable oppression'. Rather, as with Scheidt *et al.* (1999), she advocates recognition of the ups and downs of ageing in order to understand how ordinary older people 'get on with life'.

Such representations of ageing reflect wider public images in which a preoccupation with 'new fitness' has reached 'obsessive proportions' creating a powerful illusion of personal growth and fulfilment which is never quite attainable (Williams 2000). Few of us are immune from such pressures, as evidenced for example by the increase in eating disorders, the obsession with dieting and the constant media images of 'beautiful' people. Many such images are of course gendered, with women being particularly targeted. Most of us, however, can resist such images and find important sources of self-esteem from elsewhere. For others this is not so easy. Strident criticisms have come from the disability movement highlighting the 'physicality' of notions such as rehabilitation (Oliver 1993) and the deleterious effects of the constant promotion of normative criteria about physical ability as indicators of success, resulting in an 'incessant and unquestioning search for the Holy Grail of normality' (Swain and French 1998). The unquestioning adoption of independence and autonomy as policy goals for older people could result in the oldest and frailest members of society being effectively excluded from main stream policy (Dalley 2000).

Although this may yet be some way off as Nolan (Chapter 4) noted community and primary care services appear to be developing in two broad directions: those that seek to prevent or delay ill-health and disability and those aiming to promote quality of life and engagement in the community (Prophet 1998; Joseph Rowntree Foundation 1999). The evidence suggests that due to the pressure to produce quantifiable results, services place primary emphasis on the former. This is consistent with Kane's (1999) analysis that while policy makers may subscribe, in principle, to goals such as enhanced social and psychological well-being and the promotion of a meaningful life, in reality resources are targeted on more tangible and easily achievable outcomes.

This seems contrary to the notion of person-centred care which, as has been noted throughout various chapters in this book, is now writ large in the policy, practice and academic literatures. As with an integrated policy framework, however, this remains an ambition to be achieved.

From policy to practice to person-centred care

If there are a number of inconsistencies and a lack of overall clarity in policy statements for older people, recent reports, reinforced by the various reviews which comprise this book, have identified considerable variations and tensions in the quality of care older people receive. These have already been rehearsed in the relevant chapters but are perhaps typified in the case of assessment. It is widely acknowledged that assessment is the key to good practice (Audit Commission 1997; Health Advisory Service 1997; Audit Commission 1999, 2000), yet serious deficiencies in current practice were identified by all the contributors. While a number of those are attributable to lack of clear guidelines, inconsistent interpretation of policy and regional variations, lack of the relevant knowledge and skills and stereotypical attitudes among practitioners also figured prominently.

In the absence of comprehensive assessment care is compromised, not only in quality but also potentially in terms of basic competency and safety. This is manifest across the range of care environments and client groups considered in this book and raises issues about the technical adequacy of care and services. Although resource constraints are a factor, limited knowledge and skills relating to the care needs of older, and particularly vulnerable older, people are compounded by the continued denigration of so-called basic (we prefer 'fundamental' (Davies *et al.* 1999)) care.

This seems particularly ironic given the emphasis now accorded the notions of person-centred care and the avowed intention to ensure that the real experiences of service users drive quality initiatives in both the health and social services (Department of Health 1997a, 1998a, 1998b; Hutton 1999). This calls for a reconsideration of the basis of person-centred care. This cannot be divorced from an analysis of care itself, which is widely recognized as a slippery and contested concept (Atkinson 1998; Brechin 1998a, 1998b; Davies 1998). Certainly as Brechin (1998a) notes, care has been the subject of considerable debate in the policy, practice and academic literatures, but a consensus as to a definition remains elsewhere. This is not surprising given the diversity of caring circumstances but Brechin (1998a, 1998b) stresses the need to establish some common ground and identify core principles to act as a basis for action. She argues that an understanding of care must account for the balance between independence, interdependence and dependence, with good care celebrating difference while facilitating empowerment. Fundamentally she believes that care must take due account of the perspectives of all parties involved, recognizing power differentials and incorporating the importance of mediation and negotiation processes. This is particularly true of assessments in which older people and carers still play a subordinate role to that of professionals (Hardy *et al.* 1999).

Achieving improvements means accommodating the subjective experiences of those giving and receiving care in order to capture and accentuate feelings of reciprocity (Atkinson 1998). Atkinson (1998) argues that the need to feel special and valued is universal, and this is true of all those in caring relationships. Essentially therefore caring, in all its manifestations, has to be valued and accorded status (Adams *et al.* 1998; Davies 1998). This is often not the case as noted in Chapter 2, with an increasing divergence between technical as opposed to basic (fundamental) care. At a time when person-centred care is promoted so actively, Dalley (2000) contends that the delivery of care is becoming increasingly task-focused with the personal and humane qualities being 'singularly absent'. This was reinforced by the Audit Commission (1999) report on district nursing services which lamented the growing focus on technological care to the relative exclusion of personal care. Yet as this report noted, these latter elements are extremely important to patients, particularly older patients (see Chapter 4).

Treatment without care is poor and often ineffective treatment (Fitzgerald 1999) and the importance of combining proficient technical care, considerate basic (fundamental) care and good interpersonal care has been a consistent theme throughout this volume. In combination these elements elevate safe care to good or even excellent care (Davies *et al.* 1999), and it is such care that is widely regarded by older people and their family carers. A useful analogy here is that relating to reliability and validity in research. A measure may be reliable in terms of consistent performance but unless it is valid, that is measuring the right variable, it is of limited use. Reliability is therefore a necessary but not a sufficient condition for a good measure. Similarly technically competent care is a necessary but not a sufficient condition for high quality care, which must also incorporate a consideration of interpersonal dynamics and personal meanings. This latter consideration is an essential component of high quality care from the perspective of older people and their carers, attention to which is necessary to sustain feelings of self worth.

Kendig and Brooke (1999) suggest that while policy focuses largely on populations, care is primarily concerned with the 'preferences, resources and situations of individuals'. Therefore health professionals need to appreciate the goals that arise from the personal experiences and interpretations of older people who, they argue, use two main criteria to define the quality of home care they receive:

- Adequacy – is it sufficient for its purpose?
- Affirmation – of their unique identity – good care reinforces rather than threatens their sense of who they are.

In a reconceptualization of the basis for poor care in hospital settings, Coyle (1999) provided a remarkably similar framework, arguing that dissatisfaction is not a useful concept and suggesting that the notion of 'personal identity threat' more adequately captures deficient care from a patient's perspective. Coyle argues that personal identity is threatened by care which dehumanizes patients by failing to accord them value and respect their subjective experiences; disempowers patients by limiting their ability to exert control; and devalues the patient as a person. According to Coyle (1999), practitioners must be particularly sensitive to issues relating to patient's feelings of personal worth and value.

To provide good care the recipient has in some way to 'matter' and there is a need to 'value the person in the present with all their disabilities and restrictions' (Adams *et al.* 1998). Equally important is that both the care given and the caregiver are also valued and matter (Adams *et al.* 1998; Davies 1998). This is increasingly rare in health and social care, particularly, as Davies (Chapter 5) notes, in already devalued environments such as care homes where the work itself is the subject of 'multiple negative statuses' (Adams *et al.* 1998).

For Davies (1998) good care involves 'committed attending' to the recipient so that the outcomes of care are important. This means getting close to the person, whether the caring relationships is family or formal. Davies (1998) divides care into three elements:

- Caregiving – provided by family carers. This is cast primarily within a moral framework, with relatively little attention given to the type or level of skill required.
- Care-work – that care provided by unqualified and often untrained individuals. This, Davies (1998) believes, has low status which belies the skills involved and ignores the therapeutic potential of relationships.
- Professional care – based on a scientifically grounded and thorough training.

Despite the higher status of the latter relative to the other two, Davies (1998) contends that the value accorded to professional care is limited by its gendered nature and the hegemony of masculine values such as independence and autonomy which still exert the major influence in health care, even within the policies of New Labour and the Third Way.

This conclusion leads Davies (1998) to appeal for a revaluation of caring and attention to the 'urgent intellectual task' of bringing competence and caring into a new alignment. As has been suggested at various points throughout this book, and reinforced within this chapter, achieving this new alignment requires certain conditions to come together:

- Caring, in all its manifestations has to be accorded value and status. This includes technical, basic (fundamental) and interpersonal aspects. As noted by Nolan in Chapter 3, the delivery of 'hands on' care usually provides the main context in which interpersonal care is enacted. The delicate balance needed was eloquently captured by Seymour and Hanson (Chapter 6) who note that 'intersubjective enhancement of personhood through the sensitive delivery of basic care is possible'. As Dargie *et al.* (1999) conclude in their consideration of policy futures in the NHS, there has to be a proper valuation of care. There is a need to recognize the power differentials within caring situations and to appreciate that good care accommodates the perspectives of all parties involved so that none is disadvantaged. As Brechin (1998b) notes, care comprises interpersonal relationships which impact on the identity and sense of self of everyone involved. Good care should therefore reinforce rather than detract from personal identity (Coyle 1999; Kendig and Brooke 1999). This is as true of those giving care as of those receiving it. Giving care can be difficult, onerous and stressful as the extensive literature on family care attests, but it is also often satisfying (see Nolan *et al.* 1996a; Grant *et al.* 1998). This was accurately reflected by Grant in his consideration of the needs of older people with learning disabilities and the importance of recognizing the experience and analytic ability of older carers in order better to understand the resilience they so clearly demonstrate.

- There is a pressing need to articulate more clearly how 'care-work' (Davies 1998) can be satisfying and rewarding, particularly in continuing care environments and increasingly in the community. As Grant (Chapter 8) highlights care outcomes are enhanced where there is a 'development orientated' attitude among care staff, with Davies (Chapter 5) vividly describing the need to consider how older people, staff and family carers can work together to provide paths to new and improved quality of life and quality of care.

Easterbrook (1999) believes that what is required is person-centred care delivered by person-centred staff who are well motivated, well trained and who value their work. However, for people to value their work the work they do has to be valued, not only generally but also by those in receipt of care. For example, as Ingvad and Olsson (1999) point out, home carers need to feel appreciated and valued for the skills they have. This means sharing personal experiences between caregiver and care-receiver to build a relationship of confidence and trust based on congruent expectations. This sort of understanding is difficult to achieve unless there is continuity of relationship, yet this is so often compromised by the fragmented way in which services are delivered.

Reducing power differentials means recognizing and valuing differing forms of 'expertise' so that none is privileged above the other. Professional carers must therefore value the expertise that older people and family carers possess but this does not mean devaluing the central role of the 'outsider' expert. It must be appreciated therefore that an empowered client or carer is potentially very threatening to professional carers.

A return to paternalism within health care is neither desirable nor possible (Barnes 1999), but as Barnes notes, genuine involvement requires a considerable investment in organizational development and the skills and attitudes of staff. What is lacking, it seems to us, is a framework within which new relationships can be negotiated which provides a vehicle that unites the perspective of all those involved. Without this, person-centred care has about as much chance of success as seamless care. Williams *et al.* (1999) for instance in exploring the introduction of a person-centred philosophy into a mental health team highlight how this challenges the basis for relationships, with neither an 'expert-lay model' or one based on friendship being appropriate. This can erode staff confidence, which is often further threatened by empowered clients who are likely to be critical of the care they receive.

Similarly Allen (2000) has considered the impact of 'expert' carers in acute hospital settings. In contrast to the more traditional carer role of either visitor or helper, expert carers, with their strong sense of needing to advocate for the patient, destabilize the status quo. In such a situation both nurses and carers claim the right to 'know the patient' and in exerting this right, Allen (2000) argues that a battle for supremacy can result; this is potentially highly destructive.

However, taking Liaschenko's (1997) arguments (see Chapter 2) we would contend that both parties 'know the patient' – albeit in different but no less important ways. Indeed in this context were it not for the existence of a 'patient', professional and family carers would have no reason to meet. It is the existence of the 'patient' (an ill person in need of health care) that creates the relationship and this calls for a blending of case knowledge and personal knowledge. Such knowledge is not in competition, but bringing it together requires a 'reconfiguring' of expertise (Tang and Anderson 1999).

In exploring the relationship between chronically ill people and professionals, Tang and Anderson (1999) contend that both have 'agency', that is the right to exercise free will, and that neither should usurp the agency of the other. However, in certain circumstances agency may be willingly 'handed over'. So for example in new and uncertain or emergency situations 'agency' is handed over, either knowingly or by default, to professional carers. However the ultimate aim should be to have agency shared and negotiated, with the relative responsibility of assuming 'expert' status varying. Coyle (1999) in her analysis of personal identity threats in health care considers that while temporarily handing over of responsibility to professionals is not perceived as a threat, having responsibility wrest away certainly is.

The delicate skills of negotiation and mediation necessary to good care (Brechin 1998b) are even more essential when considering the situation of vulnerable older people who require substantial and often continuing support. The interaction styles suggested by Cox and Dooley (1996) relating to family caring relationships seem useful here. They described the following three styles:

- positive and proactive
- passive and accepting
- angry, negative and demanding.

The first and preferred style is facilitated when both the older person and carer value each other, and recognize and respond to each other's needs. This is analogous to the reciprocal care described by Nolan *et al.* (1996a). Too often, however, a passive and accepting or angry and negative style result from a failure of one or both parties to reflect on the needs and requirements of the other (Cox and Dooley 1996).

Nay (1999) argues that most professional care is still predicated on the basis of 'benevolent oppression', that is care 'infused with kindness but that patronises elderly persons and removes their adult rights and personhood'. If such care is to be improved there needs to be a more coherent and clearly articulated therapeutic rationale for working with older people which promotes a positive and proactive style of interaction by providing sources of satisfaction for all those involved.

An integrative approach to person-centred care

Although they have been voiced for some time calls for greater integration have recently increased from all quarters. Politicians talk of breaking down the 'Berlin Wall' between service agencies, academics advocate for a social policy relevant to an 'ageing society' rather than one focused simply on older people (Bernard and Phillips 2000) and, when asked, practitioners and older people themselves voice their concerns about fragmented, inconsistent and often inadequate support and care (Easterbrook 1999; Farrell *et al.* 1999). Integration is required at every level from government departments (Bernard and Phillips suggest a 'Ministry of Ageing'), through commissioners and providers of services to individual professions. Most importantly of all, however, there needs to be an integrated compact at the interpersonal level between these involved in the giving and receiving of care. There is, as Davies reflects in Chapter 5, a need to 'build bridges'.

Organizational change is clearly mandated but as noted in relation to the new quality agenda for the NHS innovation is not simply about 'ticking checklists – it is about changing thinking' (Department of Health 1998a). The bridges that we build therefore need to be intellectual and philosophical as well as concrete. In considering the ethical and moral implications of the growing health inequalities in the UK and the increasing tensions that will be raised by the therapeutic potential created by new health technologies, Evans (1999) calls for more prominence to be given to 'communitarian' values that recognize interdependence at a societal and community level. In the same 'policy futures' exercise Pahl (1999) argues that there is also a need better to understand people's 'micro-social' worlds, believing that it is feelings of self-worth and of being valued which 'bear so heavily' on health. Consistent with Evans (1999) he also acknowledges the importance of action at a societal level:

> It may be that relatively modest goals, such as encouraging and enabling stronger social support through personal communities and training more and better paid nurses, will do more for the health of Britain than other seemingly more dramatic measures. Building a more secure and trusting society cannot be achieved easily or quickly. In some ways it is a utopian concept. However the growth of a more stressful, competitive, unequal consumerist society does not do much good for the overall health of Britain. In the same way that people are becoming more aware of a holistic approach to their individual bodies, this could provide the basis for an encouraging and more holistic and balanced approach to society.
>
> (Pahl 1999: 22)

These are sentiments that we endorse entirely and, for us, a more holistic approach to the needs of vulnerable older people and their carers requires a reconceptualization of the bases for 'successful' ageing. This must recognize fully the importance of preventive, curative and restorative interventions but must not consign to failure those individuals who cannot aspire to such goals, nor the people, whether family or professional, who provide care and support.

Bengston *et al.* (1997) contend that gerontology as a discipline is 'data rich but theory poor'. In other words there are many 'facts' but less in the way of coherent approaches to explaining or understanding the empirical information we possess. However, as various contributions to this volume have highlighted, even basic empirical data are deficient in important areas, especially about the needs of older people with mental health problems, and older people from ethnic minority groups or those with learning disabilities. Clearly there is a need for more research but importantly also for more coherent theory building (Harper 2000) for as Poon and Gueldner (1999) stress in reflecting on the International Year of Older Persons, there is still much to learn about how 'personal meanings affect the quality, direction, satisfactions and goals of our lives'.

Personal meanings are central to an enhanced understanding as, despite the diversity of the literature consulted for this volume and the disparate constituencies comprising the review, subjective perceptions emerged as essential determinants of what constitutes a 'good life' in older age (Nilsson *et al.* 1998). Moreover such personal meanings also influence the way that care is interpreted, and the difficulties and satisfactions that care occasions whether for family carers, care-workers or professional carers. Therefore if we are to promote and successfully implement person-centred care, there is a need for some form of framework by which we can begin to explore the dimensions of such care and probe its dynamic and reciprocal nature.

There is growing recognition that 'quality', whether it be of 'life' or of 'care', hinges largely upon perceptual and subjective influences (see Chapter 1 in particular). It is no longer adequate to rely on indicators which 'lose the human being' (Kivnick and Murray 1997); there is therefore a need to move beyond 'statistical sophistication' (Bowling 1995a). Redfern (1999) suggests that we should attempt 'analytic generalisability' in synthesizing concepts which share similar meanings. Although some might object to the term 'generalisability' few, other than the most deconstructed of post-modernists, would negate the benefits of a more integrated theoretical framework.

In elaborating upon person-centred care it is our belief that any framework must be sensitive enough to account for individual variation; afford a degree of specificity so that meaningful empirical indicators of key concepts can be identified; and be relevant to disparate groups of people who both receive or provide care. Moreover in addition to facilitating new theoretical insights, a framework should be easily accessible conceptually (it should resonate with those to whom it is meant to apply) and be capable of practical application. As Brechin (1998a) suggests in exploring the core attributes of care, it is important not to get lost in the realm of abstract speculation. Consistent with Seymour and Hanson (Chapter 6) we support entirely Kitwood and Bredin's (1992a) thesis about the value of coherent theory to the enhancement of practice, for in its absence practice is relatively 'powerless at the clinical, pedagogical and political levels. A thorough theorisation provides awareness, a sense of value and a basis for concerted action'.

Although we are yet some way off a fully coherent theory we believe that we are in a position to begin to articulate a framework which elaborates some of the important dimensions of person-centred care and also illustrates how these might be achieved. This should provide for greater awareness and a sense of value, as well as a fledgling basis for more concentrated action.

In Chapter 1 we briefly outlined a framework originally suggested by Nolan (1997) as a means of providing a greater sense of therapeutic direction for staff working within continuing care settings. This comprised six senses: security, belonging, continuity, purpose, fulfilment and significance which Nolan (1997) argued were relevant both to older people and those providing care. This framework was utilized by Davies *et al.* (1999) in their study exploring good practice in the acute hospital care of older people and the results provided empirical support for its major constituents, although a sense of fulfilment was changed to a sense of achievement as this was seen as more meaningful. Importantly, the study also identified numerous ways in which each sense might be achieved (see Chapter 3 for a brief account and Davies *et al.* 1999 for full details).

On the basis of the reviews completed for this volume, and further empirical work (Davies in Chapter 5, Seymour and Hanson in Chapter 6) we would contend that the senses have more widespread relevance and application for older people across settings and for both family and formal carers. While we are not yet able to claim 'analytic generalisability' there is a high degree of 'theoretical convergence' between the senses framework and the major themes which emerged repeatedly at various points throughout this book. Furthermore the results of a number of other recent empirical studies can meaningfully be accommodated within the senses framework.

In Table 9.1 we map both existing theories/conceptualizations and empirical results on to the senses framework, together with an indication of where in this volume a more complete description can be found. In this table concepts which we believe relate to similar phenomena and empirical results which reinforce elements of the framework are compared to the relevant senses.

A consideration of Table 9.1 suggests considerable convergence and provides further theoretical and empirical support for the senses. Of most interest are the empirical data. Apart from the work of Davies *et al.* (1999), which explicitly used the senses framework, the results of the focus groups exploring community-based services with older and disabled people, carers and professionals conducted by Easterbrook (1999) and Farrell *et al.* (1999) can be meaningfully interpreted in terms of the senses, as indeed can the conclusions of the detailed study by Redfern and Norman (1999) which highlighted the parameters of good quality care in acute hospitals as perceived by patients and nurses.

As a result of the above studies and the reviews completed for this book, a more complete recounting of the senses as we currently conceive them is presented in Table 9.2.

Interestingly ongoing empirical work on the AGEIN project (see Introduction) is also demonstrating the utility of the senses in understanding student nurses' experience of working with older people and what they perceive to be a good learning environment. To date fourteen focus groups have been completed with well over a hundred informants generating large volumes of data. These data have yet to be subjected to a complete analysis and results discussed briefly below must be considered as interim. However, strong support for the 'senses' is emerging, together with a growing number of indicators as to how they might be achieved. For example students want to feel safe and secure on their ward placements and to be made to feel a member of the ward team (belonging). Continuity figures in a number of ways, highlighting the importance of having a mentor/supervisor with whom students can work regularly throughout their placements. It is important for students to be more than a 'pair of hands' and it is apparent that good ward placements allow them to engage in hands on care which stretches their ability (purpose) but within known parameters under careful unobtrusive observation (security) in order that

Table 9.1 Supporting the senses

	Theoretical frameworks				Service delivery				
	Steverink et al. 1998	Nilsson et al. 1998	Renwick and Brown 1996	Liaschenko 1997	Redfern and Norman 1999	Davies et al. 1999	Easterbrook 1999; Farrell et al. 1999	Bowsher 1994	Davies (this volume)
	Chapter 1	Chapter 1	Chapter 1	Chapter 2	Chapter 3	Chapter 3	Chapter 4	Chapter 5	Chapter 5
Security	Comfort (physical well-being)			Space	Keep promises; trust/confidence; monitor care	Visibility of staff; access to 'experts' as needed	Confidence in staff, competent and safe care		Reduce vulnerability/powerlessness
Belonging	Affection (social well-being)	Personal relationships	Belonging	Space	Homely ward atmosphere; use of affection and humour	Recognize important relationships with other patients; treated as family	Person-centred care delivered by person-centred workers; focus on interpersonal relationships	Develop/maintain positive social networks/climates	Create a sense of community
Continuity		Positive links between past and present	Being	Temporality	Maintenance of important routines; continuity of care	Named/team nursing; post-discharge follow-up	Single point of contact; continuity of carer; integrated services; understanding of life history	Generate interesting stories about lives	Maintain links with family/community
Purpose	Stimulation (physical well-being)	Activity	Becoming	Agency	Provide activity to reduce boredom	Mutually agreed goals	Clarity of goals and purpose	Develop competencies	Shared activities to create a community
Achievement	Behavioural confirmation (social well-being)	Activity	Becoming	Agency	Opportunities to achieve goals	Regular feedback on progress, being included in review	Involve older people	Attain important/valued goals	Maintain identity
Significance	Status (social well-being)	Strong personal beliefs	Being – psychological and spiritual identity		Reinforce identity and personhood	Equity of access to care; fully involved in care	Listen to expertise and voice; value older people	Experience satisfaction and positive affect	Maintain identity

Table 9.2 The six senses in the context of caring relationships

A sense of security
- For older people Attention to essential physiological and psychological needs, to feel safe and free from threat, harm, pain and discomfort. To receive competent and sensitive care.
- For staff To feel free from physical threat, rebuke or censure. To have secure conditions of employment. To have the emotional demands of work recognized and to work within a supportive but challenging culture.
- For family carers To feel confident in knowledge and ability to provide good care (To do caring well – Schumacher *et al.* 1998) without detriment to personal well-being. To have adequate support networks and timely help when required. To be able to relinquish care when appropriate.

A sense of continuity
- For older people Recognition and value of personal biography; skilful use of knowledge of the past to help contextualize present and future. Seamless, consistent care delivered within an established relationship by known people.
- For staff Positive experience of work with older people from an early stage of career, exposure to good role models and environments of care. Expectations and standards of care communicated clearly and consistently.
- For family carers To maintain shared pleasures/pursuits with the care-recipient. To be able to provide competent standards of care, whether delivered by self or others, to ensure that personal standards of care are maintained by others, to maintain involvement in care across care environments as desired/appropriate.

A sense of belonging
- For older people Opportunities to maintain and/or form meaningful and reciprocal relationships, to feel part of a community or group as desired.
- For staff To feel part of a team with a recognized and valued contribution, to belong to a peer group, a community of gerontological practitioners.
- For family carers To be able to maintain/improve valued relationships, to be able to confide in trusted individuals to feel that you are not 'in this alone'.

A sense of purpose
- For older people Opportunities to engage in purposeful activity facilitating the constructive passage of time, to be able to identify and pursue goals and challenges, to exercise discretionary choice.
- For staff To have a sense of therapeutic direction, a clear set of goals to which to aspire.
- For family carers To maintain the dignity and integrity, well being and 'personhood' of the care recipient, to pursue (re)constructive/reciprocal care (Nolan *et al.* 1996a).

A sense of achievement
- For older people Opportunities to meet meaningful and valued goals, to feel satisfied with one's efforts, to make a recognized and valued contribution, to make progress towards therapeutic goals as appropriate.
- For staff To be able to provide good care, to feel satisfied with one's efforts, to contribute towards therapeutic goals as appropriate, to use skills and ability to the full.
- For family carers To feel that you have provided the best possible care, to know you've 'done your best', to meet challenges successfully, to develop new skills and abilities.

A sense of significance
- For older people To feel recognized and valued as a person of worth, that one's actions and existence are of importance, that you 'matter'.
- For staff To feel that gerontological practice is valued and important, that your work and efforts 'matter'.
- For family carers To feel that one's caring efforts are valued and appreciated, to experience an enhanced sense of self.

Source: Developed from Nolan *et al.* 1996a, Nolan 1997 and Davies *et al.* 1999

they can fully meet their formal learning objectives as well as their own personal learning agendas (achievement). In such circumstances students feel that they are making a genuine and meaningful contribution to patient care (significance) (Brown *et al.* 2000).

The above represents only an initial and superficial consideration of the data and more detailed analysis will provide further insights into the robustness and relevance of the senses framework as well as elaborating upon its various dimensions. It is already apparent that the 'senses' interact in subtle and dynamic ways and that their relative importance shifts over time. For example during early ward experiences, neophyte students place considerable importance on security and belonging, rather than purpose and achievement. As they progress and become more confident and competent, security and belonging, although still essential, are displaced relative to purpose and achievement. Students want to be able to demonstrate and refine their emerging skill base. Interestingly as qualification approaches and work as a staff nurse comes ever closer, security and belonging rise once more to the forefront (Brown *et al.* 2000).

We anticipate that such variation both over time and according to the environment and context of care will occur when the senses framework is applied to older people and family and professional carers. For example a sense of belonging was important to staff in the Davies *et al.* (1999) study on acute hospital wards and was manifest in a number of ways including being a part of the nursing and multidisciplinary teams, with the metaphor of 'a family' often being used to describe good wards. Conversely in the private sector such a sense of belonging can often be more difficult to achieve due to the lower numbers of qualified staff and the relatively few opportunities to work with colleagues on a regular basis.

Similarly the way in which the senses might be achieved and their relative emphasis will vary for older people according to the environment of care. In an acute hospital ward, patients still value a sense of belonging and relationships with other patients are very important in achieving this (see Davies *et al.* 1999), although such belonging is transient because discharge, ideally home, is the ultimate aim. A delicate balance therefore has to be struck between creating a feeling of belonging while also recognizing the temporary nature of relationships. On the other hand 'belonging' within a care home environment has differing temporal dimensions and, as Davies (Chapter 5) highlights, it is essential to create a sense of community.

While we feel that the major dimensions in the emergent 'senses' framework are robust, there remains much to explore further. The senses reflect important parameters of good care and capture some of the dimensions of 'person-centredness'. Certainly in their absence, care is often manifestly deficient as evidenced for instance in the telling data recounted by Seymour and Hanson (Chapter 6). Equally the same chapter suggests how the presence of the 'senses' can enhance care.

In addition to elaborating upon some of the empirical referents of person-centred care the senses also have the potential to provide greater therapeutic direction for staff, with work in continuing care contexts providing a fine example. Such work often lacks a clear purpose, resulting in 'aimless residual care' (Evers 1991) or the adoption of spurious and often abusive goals such as the 'lounge standard patient' (Lee-Treweek 1994). Successive studies since the early 1960s have recounted the difficulties of providing sustained high quality care for vulnerable groups of older people; things are unlikely to improve until staff feel that their work has a purpose and is accorded value and significance. Moreover as person-centred care requires staff to invest of themselves in older people, there is a need for adequate support structures when, for example, an older person dies (see Nolan and Keady 1996).

These are just a few examples of the potential applications of the senses framework. The next stage of the AGEIN project involves further testing and refinement of the framework with key reference groups of older people and family and formal caregivers, in order to elaborate upon our current understanding.

Envoi

As we go to press the National Science Framework (NSF) for older people is imminent and while its contents are as yet unknown, person-centredness is likely to lie at the heart of its recommendations (Philp *et al.* 2000). Central to the success of the NSF will be staff who possess the necessary knowledge, skills and competences to care for older people (Hutton 1999) and, we would add, are able to make manifest the high ideals underpinning person-centred care. This, as noted by others, will mean reorientating both policy and practice towards individual experience (Department of Health 1997a; Dargie *et al.* 1999).

However, notwithstanding the importance of individual experience, quality of care is unlikely to be optimally enhanced until communitarian values and practices (Evans 1999) figure more prominently. These must be reflected in broader and more holistic measures of quality (Dargie *et al.* 1999) and embedded within the educational preparation of all practitioners. Well-motivated and well-educated personnel who value their work are essential prerequisites to improved practice (Easterbrook 1999) but unfortunately work with older people is still accorded little value or status (Easterbrook 1999) and is often the least preferred career option (Stevens 1999). Paradoxically, despite work with older people necessitating intellectual and interpersonal skills of the highest order it is generally perceived to be relatively undemanding: not requiring the level of expertise essential in more technologically orientated aspects of care (Nay and Closs 1999).

Nay and Closs (1999) highlight the relative neglect of gerontology in professional curricula, and the dearth of positive role models and practice environments to which practitioners are exposed during their training. This must change as new ways of working and quality initiatives must be 'owned' by staff, who are motivated to meet future agendas (Dargie *et al.* 1999). As we noted in the Introduction, this volume is the product of a particular research study aimed specifically, but certainly not exclusively, at improving the education of nurses in order that they provide improved services to older people and their carers. It is our hope that the framework we have presented, incomplete and emerging as it is, will help to realize not only this aim but also to stimulate debate and to promote genuine partnerships between all those involved in addressing the needs of an ageing society.

APPENDIX

Study methodology

The AGEIN Project comprises a number of distinct but overlapping and complementary phases intended to help identify a knowledge base for practice with older people and their family carers. Phases 1 and 2 of the project run concurrently with the existing volume being the interim product of Phase 1. This book is based on an extensive review of the available literature in six key areas of practice with older people, augmented by new data collected in a number of these areas:

- Acute/rehabilitative care
- Primary care
- Continuing care
- Older people with mental health problems
- Older people with learning disabilities
- Palliative care and older people.

It is important to highlight at this point that extensive volumes of data have been collected to date, and continue to be collected. However, this volume does not draw primarily on the data but is rather the product of the review analysis and synthesis process.

The intention of the review was to identify areas of commonality and contrast in the above areas that might begin to form the basis for an epistemology of practice with older people. The identification of literature sources was rigorous and the guiding principle behind the mechanics of the review was that it should be systematic, explicit and reproducible (Nolan *et al.* 1997). In order to produce a synthesis of knowledge across six distinct areas of practice with older people, it was important that the review was carried out in a consistent manner across these boundaries. This would also allow the review to be regularly updated. A wide range of bibliographic sources was consulted in order to identify literature emerging from a range of professional and academic disciplines (Table A.1).

Work produced during the period 1988–98 provided the initial focus for the search. Key references identified from the retrieved sources which were published before this period were also included and the review was regularly updated as new items entered the public domain.

Table A.1 Bibliographic sources consulted for the review

Cinahl	–	the Cumulative Index to Nursing and Allied Health Literature provides coverage of the literature related to nursing and allied health
Medline	–	encompasses information from Index Medicus, Index to Dental Literature and International Nursing as well as other sources of coverage
Psychlit	–	covers international literature on psychology and related fields
Bids	–	ISI service provides access to four bibliographic databases supplied by the Institute for Scientific Information, covering scientific and technical information, social science, arts and humanities; we searched the social science database
AgeInfo	–	the database from the Centre for Policy on Ageing
HMIC	–	the Health Management Information Consortium brings together three complete bibliographic databases covering UK and overseas health management and related topics; the three databases included are the Department of Health Library, the Nuffield Institute for Health database and the King's Fund database

Search terms were identified by chapter authors for each of the discrete areas. When these were collated, it became apparent that many of the themes and concepts were common to all six areas and these became core terms which were relevant across the entire review. Search terms specific to each field of practice were also subsequently identified (Table A.2).

This approach initially identified in excess of 22,000 references. The majority of these items were academic papers in peer reviewed journals, with books and reports contributing approximately 5 per cent of the total. The abstract for each item was scrutinized and key themes and concepts identified. Material that was obviously not relevant to the focus of the review was eliminated at this stage. Following this initial classification, each abstract was examined a second time and an attempt was made to prioritize references in order to produce a more manageable volume of literature for retrieval and closer scrutiny. For example, those that appeared to represent service user views and professional views and those representing rigorous reviews of the literature, or which claimed to provide new theoretical insights, were given a higher priority. This process resulted in the identification of approximately 200 to 300 items for each field. These items were then retrieved, reviewed and grouped thematically to provide a structure for each chapter.

In reviewing each reference a broad three-stage iterative process was followed. Initially, each reference was read independently and a set of notes made identifying and summarizing key themes. Subsequently, the notes from this first order analysis were scrutinized in detail so as to distil the core attributes of the key themes. Finally, comparisons were made within and between themes to explore the conceptual links and achieve an element of synthesis. For a detailed account of the principles underpinning both the relevance of literature and the subsequent analyses see Nolan *et al.* (1997).

Following the review process and the identification of the 'senses' framework (see Table 9.2) the next stage of the project is to expose this emerging framework to more detailed empirical scrutiny in order to further elaborate upon its dimensions and

Table A.2 Core and specific search terms

	Mike Nolan	Liz Hanson	Gordon Grant	Sue Davies	Janet Nolan	John Keady
Field of study	Acute and rehabilitative care	Palliative care	Learning disabilities	Continuing care	Primary care	Mental health
Core terms	Ethnic group and ethnicity Quality of life Communication Needs and needs assessment Nursing care Carers Models Discharge Services					
Specific terms	Rehabilitation Rehabilitation nursing Acute care	End-of-life care and decision making Long-term care Quality of life Palliative care Terminal care Hospice care Death Bereavement	Learning disorders Learning difficulty Learning disability Developmental disabilities Intellectual disability Mental retardation Rational processes disorder Mental health services	Continuing care Nursing homes Retirement centres Residential homes Residential care	Primary health care Community health services Community health nursing District nursing Health visiting Practice nursing	Mental health Community mental health services Dementia Mental processes Schizophrenia Late-onset paraphrenia Anxiety disorders Depression Alcohol misuse HIV

provide a more detailed examination of its attributes. This will involve older people and family carers as well as professionals (primarily, but not exclusively, nurses). The intention is to identify more clearly those aspects of person-centred care that appear to be most relevant to achieving high quality care for older people in a range of care environments.

Complementing the above process is another phase of data collection, which explores the educational experience of nurses at both pre- and post-registration levels. This phase involves a combination of in-depth interviews, focus groups and postal surveys of student nurses and qualified practitioners. The majority of data collection is taking place in four case study sites but these data will be augmented by a national survey of qualified practitioners together with surveys of university students and members of the general public in order to be able to compare the perceptions of nurses with a more general population.

Phase 3 of the study will comprise a synthesis of the products of 1 and 2 in order to identify how the study results might best inform the education of nurses and older practitioners. It is therefore important to recognize that this work constitutes an interim product of the AGEIN study. Data collection and analysis is currently ongoing and the study is due for completion in September 2001.

Bibliography

Abrams, R.C., Teresi, J.A. and Butin, D.N. (1992) Depression in nursing home residents, *Clinics in Geriatric Medicine*, 8(2): 309–22.

Adams, A. and Wilson, A. (1996) Accommodation for older people with mental health problems, *Findings: Social Care Research*, 87: 4.

Adams, J., Burrit, J. and Prickett, M. (1998) Discovering the present in stories about the past, in A. Brechin, J. Walmsley, J. Katz and S. Peace (eds) *Care Matters: Concepts, Practice and Research in Health and Social Care*. London: Sage.

Adams, T. (1989) Growth of a specialty, *Nursing Times*, 85(40): 30–2.

Adams, T. (1991) A family stress model of dementia, *Senior Nurse*, 11(2): 33–5.

Adams, T. (1994) The emotional experience of caregivers to relatives who are chronically confused: implications for community mental health nursing, *International Journal of Nursing Studies*, 31(6): 545–53.

Adams, T. (1996a) Kitwood's approach to dementia and dementia care: a critical but appreciative review, *Journal of Advanced Nursing*, 23: 948–53.

Adams, T. (1996b) Informal family caregiving to older people with dementia: research priorities for community psychiatric nursing, *Journal of Advanced Nursing*, 24: 703–10.

Adams, T. (1996c) A descriptive study of the work of community psychiatric nurses with elderly demented people, *Journal of Advanced Nursing*, 23: 1177–84.

Adams, T. (1998) The discursive construction of dementia care: implications for mental health nursing, *Journal of Advanced Nursing*, 28: 614–21.

Addington-Hall, J.M. (1998) *Reaching Out: Specialist Palliative Care for Adults with Non-Malignant Diseases*, occasional paper no. 14. London: National Council for Hospice and Specialist Palliative Care and Scottish Partnership Agency for Palliative Cancer Care.

Addington-Hall, J.M. and McCarthy, M. (1995) Regional study of care for the dying: methods and sample characteristics, *Palliative Medicine*, 9: 27–35.

Addington-Hall, J.M., Lay, M., Altmann, D. and McCarthy, M. (1995) Symptom control, communication with health professionals and hospital care of stroke patients in the last year of life, as reported by surviving family, friends and carers, *Stroke*, 26: 2242–8.

Addington-Hall, J.M., Lay, M., Altmann, D. and McCarthy, M. (1998a) Community care for stroke patients in the last year of life: results of national retrospective survey of surviving family, friends and officials, *Health and Social Care in the Community*, 6: 112–19.

Addington-Hall, J.M., Fakhoury, W. and McCarthy, M. (1998b) Specialist palliative care in non-malignant disease, *Palliative Medicine*, 12: 417–27.

Age Concern (1996) HIV, AIDS and older people, *Elders: Journal of Care and Practice*, 5(3): 5–11.

Age Concern (2000) *Turning your back on us*. London: Age Concern.

Ahmedzai, S. (1995) Palliative care for all? (editorial), *Progress in Palliative Care*, 2: 77–9.

Albert, S.M., Marks, J., Barrett, V. and Gurland, B. (1997) Home health care and quality of life of patients with Alzheimer's disease, *American Journal of Preventative Medicine*, 13(6): 63–8.

Alford, D.M. and Futrell, M. (1992) Wellness and health promotion of the elderly, *Nursing Outlook*, 40(5): 221–6.

Allen, D. (2000) Negotiating the role of expert carers on an adult hospital ward, *Sociology of Health and Illness*, 22(2): 149–71.

Allen, I., Levin, E., Siddell, M. and Vetter, N. (1983) The elderly and their informal carers, in *Elderly People in the Community: Their Service Needs*. London: HMSO.

Allison, M. and Keller, C. (1997) Physical activity in the elderly: benefits and intervention strategies, *Nurse Practitioner: American Journal of Primary Health Care*, 22(8): 53–4.

Alzheimer's Disease Society (1994) *Home Alone: Living Alone with Dementia*. London: Alzheimer's Disease Society.

Alzheimer's Disease Society (1995) *Dementia in the Community: Management Strategies for General Practice*. London: Alzheimer's Disease Society.

Alzheimer's Disease Society (1997) *No Accounting for Health: Health Commissioning for Dementia*. London: Alzheimer's Disease Society.

American Psychiatric Association (1987) *Diagnostic and Statistical Manual of Mental Disorders* (3rd edn, revised DSM-III-R). Washington, DC: American Psychiatric Association.

American Psychiatric Association (1994) *DSM-IV: Diagnostic and Statistical Manual of Mental Disorders*, 4th edn. Washington, DC: American Psychiatric Association.

Anderson, D.J. (1989) Healthy and institutionalised: health and related conditions among older persons with developmental disabilities, *Journal of Applied Gerontology*, 8(2): 228–41.

Anderson, D.J. (1993) Social inclusion of older adults with mental retardation, in E. Sutton, A.R. Factor, B.A. Hawkins, T. Heller and G.B. Seltzer (eds) *Older Adults with Developmental Disabilities: Optimizing Choice and Change*. Baltimore, MD: Paul H. Brookes.

Andrews, K. (1987) *Rehabilitation of Older Adults*. London: Edward Arnold.

Arber, S. and Gilbert, N. (1989) Transitions in caring gender, life course and the care of the elderly, in B. Bytheway, P. Allatt, T. Keil and A. Bryman (eds) *Becoming and Being Old: Sociological Approaches to Later Life*. London: Sage.

Archbold, P.G., Stewart, B.J., Greenlick, M.R. and Harvath, T.A. (1992) The clinical assessment of mutuality and preparedness in family caregivers to frail older people, in S.G. Funk, E.M. Tornquist, M.T. Champagne and A. Copp (eds) *Key Aspects of Elder Care: Managing Falls, Incontinence and Cognitive Impairment*. New York: Springer.

Armstrong-Esther, C.A., Browne, K.D. and McAfee, J.G. (1994) Elderly patients: still clean and sitting quietly, *Journal of Advanced Nursing*, 19(2): 264–71.

Aronheim, J.C. (1997) End of life issues for very elderly women: incurable and terminal illness, *Journal of the American Women's Medical Association*, 52(3): 147–51.

Arrington, D.T. (1997) Retirement communities as creative clinical opportunities, *N & HC Perspectives on Community*, 18(2): 82–5.

Ashaye, O., Mathew, G. and Dhadphale, M. (1997) A comparison of older longstay psychiatric and learning disability inpatients using the Health of the Nation Outcome Scales, *International Journal of Geriatric Psychiatry*, 12: 548–52.

Ashton, P. and Keady, J. (1999) Mental disorders of older people, in R. Newell and K. Gournay (eds) *Mental Health Nursing: an Evidence Based Approach*. Edinburgh: Churchill Livingstone.

Askham, J. (1998) Supporting caregivers of older people: an overview of problems and priorities. *Australian Journal of Ageing*, 17(1), 5–7.

Åström, S. (1986) Health care students' attitudes towards, and intention to work with, patients suffering from senile dementia, *Journal of Advanced Nursing*, 11: 651–9.

Atkinson, D. (1998) Living in residential care, in A. Brechin, J. Walmsley, J. Katz and S. Peace (eds) *Care Matters: Concepts, Practice and Research in Health and Social Care*. London: Sage.

Audit Commission (1997) *The Coming of Age: Improving Care Services for Older People*. London: Audit Commission.

Audit Commission (1999) *First Assessment: a Review of District Nursing Services in England and Wales*. London: Audit Commission.

Audit Commission (2000) *Forget Me Not: Mental Health Services for Older People*. London: Audit Commission.

Avis, M., Greening Jackson, J., Cox, K. and Miskella, C. (1999) Evaluation of a project providing community palliative care support to nursing homes, *Health and Social Care in the Community*, 7(1): 32–8.

Bach, M. and Rioux, M.H. (1996) Social well-being: a framework for quality of life research, in R. Renwick, I. Brown and M. Nagler (eds) *Quality of Life in Health Promotion and Rehabilitation: Conceptual Approaches, Issues and Applications*. Thousand Oaks, CA: Sage.

Badger, T.A. (1996) Living with depression: family members' experiences and treatment needs, *Journal of Psychosocial Nursing and Mental Health Services*, 34(1): 21–9.

Baer, E.D. and Gordon, S. (1996) Money managers are unravelling the tapestry of nursing, in S. Gordon, P. Benner and N. Noddings (eds) *Caregiving: Readings in Knowledge, Practice, Ethics and Politics*. Philadelphia, PA: University of Pennsylvania Press.

Baker, M., Fardell, J. and Jones, B. (1997) *Disability and Rehabilitation: Survey of Education Needs of Health and Social Service Professionals – The Case for Action*. London: Disability and Rehabilitation, Open Learning Project.

Baldwin, N., Harris, J. and Kelly, D. (1993) Institutionalisation: why blame the institutions?, *Ageing and Society*, 13: 69–81.

Baltes, M. and Carstensen, L.L. (1996) The process of successful ageing, *Ageing and Society*, 16(4): 397–422.

Baltes, M.M., Neumann, E.M. and Zank, S. (1994) Maintenance and rehabilitation of independence in old age: an intervention program for staff, *Psychology and Ageing*, 9(2): 179–88.

Banks, P. (1999) *Carer Support: Time for a Change of Direction*. London: King's Fund.

Barker, P.J., Reynolds, W. and Stevenson, C. (1997) The human science basis of psychiatric nursing: theory and practice, *Journal of Advanced Nursing*, 25(4): 660–7.

Barker, P., Keady, J., Croom, S. *et al.* (1998) The concept of serious mental illness:

modern myths and grim realities, *Journal of Psychiatric and Mental Health Nursing*, 5(4): 247–54.

Barnard, D. (1995) Chronic illness and the dynamics of hoping, in R. Toombs, D. Barnard and E. Carson (eds) *Chronic Illness: From Experience to Policy*. Bloomington, IN: Indiana University Press.

Barnes, M. (1999) *Public Expectations: From Paternalism to Partnership, Changing Relationships in Health and Health Services*. Policy futures for UK health, no. 10. London: Nuffield Trust.

Barnes, M. and Walker, A. (1996) Consumerism versus empowerment: a principled approach to the involvement of older service users, *Policy and Politics*, 24(4): 375–93.

Barolin, G.S. (1996) Geriatric rehabilitation ('Alters-rehabilitation') – the new challenge for social medicine and science, *International Journal of Rehabilitation Research*, 19(3): 201–18.

Bartels, S.J., Horn, S., Sharkey, P. and Levine, K. (1997) Treatment of depression in older primary care patients in health maintenance organizations, *International Journal of Psychiatry in Medicine*, 27(3): 215–31.

Bartlett, H. (1993) *Nursing Homes for Elderly People: Questions of Quality and Policy*. Chur, Switzerland: Harwood.

Bartlett, H. and Burnip, S. (1998) Quality of care in nursing homes for older people: providers' perspectives and priorities, *NT Research*, 3(4): 257–68.

Beardshaw, V. (1988) *Last in the List: Community Services for People with Physical Disabilities*. London: King's Fund Institute.

Becker, G. (1994) Age bias in stroke rehabilitation – effects on adult status, *Journal of Aging Studies*, 8(3): 271–90.

Beckingham, A.C. and Watt, S. (1995) Daring to grow old: Lessons in healthy aging and empowerment, *Educational Gerontology*, 21: 479–95.

Beckmann, J. and Ditlev, G. (1992) Conceptual views on quality of life, in A. Kaplun (ed.) *Health Promotion and Chronic Illness: Discovering a New Quality of Health*. Copenhagen: WHO Regional Publications.

Beery, J.M. (1993) Control issues for residents of long-term care facilities. Unpublished PhD thesis, the Union Institute.

Bengston, V.L., Burgess, E.O. and Parrat, T.M. (1997) Theory, explanation and a third generation of theoretical development in social gerontology, *Journal of Gerontology (Social Series)*, 52(2): 572–88.

Benner, P. (1984) *From Novice to Expert: Excellence and Power in Clinical Nursing*. Menlo Park, CA: Addison-Wesley.

Benner, P. and Gordon, S. (1996) Caring practice, in S. Gordon, P. Benner and N. Noddings (eds) *Caregiving: Readings in Knowledge, Practice, Ethics and Politics*. Philadelphia, PA: University of Pennsylvania Press.

Benner, P. and Wruebel, J. (1989) *The Primary of Caring: Stress and Coping in Health and Illness*. Menlo Park, CA: Addison-Wesley.

Benner, P., Tanner, C.A. and Chesla, C.A. (1996) *Expertise in Nursing Practice: Caring, Clinical Judgement and Ethics*. New York: Springer.

Beresford, B. (1994) *Positively Parents: Caring for a Severely Disabled Child*. London: HMSO.

Bergen, A. and Labute, L. (1993) Promoting effective drug taking by elderly people in the community, in A. Dines and A. Cribb (eds) *Health Promotion Concepts and Practice*. Oxford: Blackwell Scientific Publications.

Bernard, M. and Phillips, J. (1998) Ageing in tomorrow's Britain, in M. Bernard and J. Phillips (eds) *The Social Policy of Old Age.* London: Centre for Policy on Ageing.

Bernard, M. and Phillips, J. (2000) The challenge of ageing in tomorrow's Britain, *Ageing and Society*, 20(1): 33–54.

Best, C. (1998) Caring for the individual, *Elderly Care*, 10(5): 20–4.

Bettison, J. (1988) The alternative to crisis visiting, *Health Visitor*, 61(1): 13–15.

Biedenharn, P.J. and Normoyle, J.B. (1991) Elderly community residents' reactions to the nursing home: an analysis of nursing home-related beliefs, *Gerontologist*, 31(1): 107–15.

Biegal, D.E. and Farkas, K.J. (1997) Barriers to the use of mental health services by African-American and Hispanic elderly person, *Journal of Gerontological Social Work*, 29(1): 23–44.

Bigby, C. (1997) When parents relinquish care: informal support networks of older people with intellectual disability, *Journal of Applied Research in Intellectual Disabilities*, 10(4): 333–44.

Black, D. and Bowman, C. (1997) Community institutional care for frail elderly people, *British Medical Journal*, 300: 983–6.

Blackburn, A.M. (1989) Problems of terminal care in elderly patients, *Palliative Medicine*, 3: 203–6.

Blair, C.E., Lewis, R., Vieweg, V. and Tucker, R. (1996) Group and single-subject evaluation of a programme to promote self-care in elderly nursing home residents, *Journal of Advanced Nursing*, 24(6): 1207–13.

Blaxter, M. (1976) *The Meaning of Disability.* London: Heinemann.

Blazer, D.G. (1982) *Depression in Late Life.* London: Mosby.

Bliesmer, M. and Earle, P. (1993) Research considerations: nursing home quality perceptions, *Journal of Gerontological Nursing*, 19(6): 27–34.

Bliesmer, M.M., Smayling, M., Kane, R.L. and Shannon, I. (1998) The relationship between nursing staffing levels and nursing home outcomes, *Journal of Aging and Health*, 10(3): 351–71.

Bogdan, R. and Taylor, S.J. (1989) Relationships with severely disabled people: the social construction of humanness, *Social Problems*, 36(2): 135–48.

Bogo, M. (1987) Social work practice and family systems in adaptation to homes for the aged, *Journal of Gerontological Social Work*, 1/2: 5–20.

Boland, D.L. and Sims, S.L. (1996) Family care giving at home as a solitary journey, *Image: Journal of Nursing Scholarship*, 28(1): 55–8.

Bond, J. (1997) Stroke, in I. Philp (ed.) *Outcomes Assessment for Healthcare in Elderly People.* London: Ferrand Press.

Booth, T. (1985) *Home Truths: Old People's Homes and the Outcome of Care.* Aldershot: Gower.

Bosanquet, N. (1997) New challenge for palliative care: to share its special mission with a wider audience (editorial), *British Medical Journal*, 314: 1294.

Bott, K. (1998) Improving links between hospitals and nursing homes – a practical project. Paper presented to the Annual Conference of the Relatives Association, 9 November, London.

Bowers, B.J. (1987) Intergenerational caregiving: adult caregivers and their ageing parents, *Advances in Nursing Science*, 9(2): 20–31.

Bowles, L., Oliver, N. and Stanley, S. (1995) A fresh approach, *Nursing Times*, 91(1): 40–1.

Bowling, A. (1991) *Measuring Health: a Review of the Quality of Life Measurement Scales.* Buckingham: Open University Press.

Bowling, A. (1995a) The most important things in life: comparisons between older and younger population age groups by gender: results from a national survey of the public's judgements, *International Journal of Health Sciences*, 6(4): 169–75.

Bowling, A. (1995b) *Measuring Disease: a Review of Disease-Specific Quality of Life Measurement Scales*. Buckingham: Open University Press.

Bowling, A. (1998) Measuring health related quality of life among older people, *Aging and Mental Health*, 2(1): 5–6.

Bowling, A. and Formby, J. (1991) Nurses' attitudes to elderly people: a survey of nursing homes and elderly care wards in an inner-London health district, *Nursing Practice*, 5(1): 16–24.

Bowsher, J.E. (1994) A theoretical model of independence for nursing home elders, *Scholarly Inquiry for Nursing Practice*, 8(2): 207–24.

Bowsher, J.E. and Gerlach, M.J. (1990) Personal control and other determinants of psychological well-being in nursing home elders, *Scholarly Inquiry for Nursing Practice*, 4(2): 91–102.

Bradshaw, A. (1995) What are nurses doing to patients? A review of theories of nursing past and present, *Journal of Clinical Nursing*, 4: 81–92.

Braithwaite, V.A. (1990) *Bound to Care*. Sydney: Allen & Unwin.

Brändstädter, J. and Greve, W. (1994) The aging self: stabilising and protective processes, *Developmental Review*, 14: 52–80.

Brändstädter, J., Wentura, D. and Greve, W. (1993) Adoptive resources of the aging self: outlines of an emergent perspective, *International Journal of Behavioural Development*, 16(2): 323–49.

Brechin, A. (1998a) Introduction, in A. Brechin, J. Walmsley, J. Katz and S. Peace (eds) *Care Matters: Concepts, Practice and Research in Health and Social Care*. London: Sage.

Brechin, A. (1998b) What makes for good care?, in A. Brechin, J. Walmsley, J. Katz and S. Peace (eds) *Care Matters: Concepts, Practice and Research in Health and Social Care*. London: Sage.

Brereton, L. and Nolan, M. (2000) You do know he's had a stroke don't you? Preparation for family caregiving – the neglected dimension, *Journal of Clinical Nursing*, 9: 498–506.

Brillhart, B. and Sills, F.B. (1994) Analysis of the roles and responsibilities of rehabilitation nursing staff, *Rehabilitation Nursing*, 19(3): 145–50.

Brocklehurst, J. and Dickinson, E. (1996) Autonomy for elderly people in long-term care, *Age and Ageing*, 25(4): 329–32.

Brocklehurst, N. (1997) Clinical supervision in nursing homes, *Nursing Times*, 93(12): 48–9.

Brodaty, H. and Gresham, M. (1997) The Prince Henry Hospital dementia caregivers' training programme., *International Journal of Geriatric Psychiatry*, 12(2): 183–92.

Brooker, D., Foster, N., Banner, A., Payne, M. and Jackson, L. (1998) The efficacy of Dementia Care Mapping as an audit tool: report on a 3-year British NHS evaluation, *Aging and Mental Health*, 2(1): 60–70.

Brown, C. and Thompson, K. (1994) A quality life: searching for quality of life in residential service for elderly people, *Australian Journal on Ageing*, 13(3): 131–3.

Brown, I., Renwick, R. and Nagler, M. (1996a) The centrality of quality of life in health promotion and rehabilitation, in R. Renwick, I. Brown and M. Nagler (eds) *Quality of Life in Health Promotion and Rehabilitation: Conceptual Approaches, Issues and Applications*. Thousand Oaks, CA: Sage.

Brown, S.M., Humphry, R. and Taylor, E. (1996b) A model of the nature of family–therapist relationships: implications for education, *The American Journal of Occupational Therapy*, 51(7): 597–603.

Brown, J., Nolan, M.R. and Davies, S. (2000) *The AGEIN Project: Phase 2 Interim Report*. Submitted to English National Board for Nursing, Midwifery and Health Visiting, London, April 2000.

Bryant, E.T. (1995) Acute rehabilitation: an outcome orientated model, in P.K. Landrum, N.D. Schmidt and A.J. McLean (eds) *Outcome Orientated Rehabilitation: Principles, Strategies and Tools for Effective Program Management*. Gaithersburg, MD: Aspen.

Bryant, H. and Fernald, L. (1997) Nursing knowledge and use of restraint alternatives: acute and chronic care, *Geriatric Nursing*, 18(2): 57–60.

Buckwalter, K.C., Cusack, D., Sidles, E., Wadle, K. and Beaver, M. (1989) Increasing communication ability in aphasic/dysarthric patients, *Western Journal of Nursing Research*, 11(6): 736–47.

Buckwalter, K.C., Cusack, D., Kruckeberg, T. and Shoemaker, A. (1991) Family involvement with communication impaired residents in long-term care settings, *Applied Nursing Research*, 4(2): 77–84.

Buffman, M. and Brod, M. (1998) Humor and well-being in spouse caregivers of patients with Alzheimer's disease, *Applied Nursing Research*, 11(1): 12–18.

Burgener, S. (1994) Caregiver religiosity and well-being in dealing with Alzheimer's dementia, *Journal of Religion and Health*, 33(2): 175–89.

Burke, L. (1997) Putting Working Paper 10 into practice: education and training, *British Journal of Nursing*, 6(14): 666–70.

Burridge, R. (1988) The role of the health visitor with the elderly, *Health Visitor*, 61: 20–1.

Bury, M. (1982) Chronic illness as biographical disruption, *Sociology of Health and Illness*, 4(2): 167–82.

Bury, M. and Holme, A. (1991) *Life after Ninety*. London: Routledge.

Bycock, I. (1996) The nature of suffering and the nature of opportunity at the end of life, *Clinics in Geriatric Medicine*, 12(2): 237–52.

Callahan, D. (1987) *Setting Limits: Medical Goals in an Ageing Society*. New York: Simon and Schuster.

Campbell, J.M. and Linc, L.G. (1996) Support groups for visitors of residents in nursing homes, *Journal of Gerontological Nursing*, 22(2): 30–5, 54–5.

Carlsen, W.R., Galluzzi, K.E., Forman, L.F. and Cavalitti, T.A. (1994) Comprehensive geriatric assessment: applications for community-residing, elderly people with mental retardation/developmental disabilities, *Mental Retardation*, 32(5): 334–40.

Carpenter, I. and Calnan, M. (1997) Grey matters, *Health Services Journal*, 107: 22–3.

Carricaburu, D. and Pierret, J. (1995) From biographical disruption to biographical reinforcement: the case of HIV positive men, *Sociology of Health and Illness*, 17(1): 65–92.

Carson, R.A. (1995) Beyond respect to recognition and due regard in S.K. Toombs, D. Barnard and R.A. Carson (eds) *Chronic Illness: from Experience to Policy*. Bloomington, IN: Indiana University Press.

Cartwright, A. (1993) Dying when you're old, *Age and Ageing*, 22: 425–30.

Cartwright, A. and Seale, C.F. (1990) *The Natural History of a Survey: an Account of Methodological Issues Encountered in a Study of Life before Death*. London: King's Fund.

Cartwright, A., Hockey, L. and Anderson, J.L. (1973) *Life Before Death*. London: Routledge and Kegan Paul.

Cartwright, J.C., Archbold, P.G., Stewart, B.J. and Limandri, B. (1994) Enrichment processes in family caregiving to frail elders, *Advances in Nursing Sciences*, 17(1): 31–43.

Casey, M.S. and Holmes, C.A. (1995) The inner ache: an experiential perspective on loneliness, *Nursing Inquiry*, 2(3): 172–9.

Cassell, E.J. (1991) *The Nature of Suffering and the Goals of Medicine*. New York: Oxford University Press.

Centre for Policy on Ageing (1999) *National Required Standards for Residential and Nursing Homes for Older People*. London: Department of Health and the Welsh Office.

Challis, D. (1981) The measurement of outcome in social care of the elderly, *Journal of Social Policy*, 10(2): 179–208.

Charmaz, K. (1983) Loss of self: a fundamental form of suffering in the chronically ill, *Sociology of Health and Illness*, 5(2): 168–95.

Charmaz, K. (1987) Struggling for self: identify levels of the chronically ill, *Research in the Sociology of Health Care*, 6: 283–321.

Charmove, A.S. and Young, M.G. (1989) Surveillance evaluation for the elderly, *Health Visitor*, 62: 301–2.

Chen, K. and Snyder, M. (1996) Perception of personal control and satisfaction with care among nursing home elders, *Perspectives*, 20(2): 16–19.

Chesson, R., Macleod, M. and Massie, S. (1996) Outcome measures used in therapy departments in Scotland, *Physiotherapy*, 82(12): 673–9.

Cheston, R. and Bender, M. (1999) *Understanding Dementia: the Man with the Worried Eyes*. London: Jessica Kingsley.

Chilvers, J.R. and Jones, D. (1997) The teaching nursing homes innovation: a literature review, *Journal of Advanced Nursing*, 26(3): 463–9.

Chochinov, H.M., Wilson, K.G., Enns, M. *et al.* (1995) Desire for death in the terminally ill, *American Journal of Psychiatry*, 152: 1185–91.

Cirincoine, U.K. and Fattore, L. (1996) Improving the oral health of older adults, *Family and Community Health*, 18(4): 9–19.

Clark, C.A., Corroran, M. and Gitlin, L.N. (1994) An exploratory study of how occupational therapies develop between relationships with family caregivers, *American Journal of Occupational Therapy*, 49(7): 587–94.

Clark, D. (1997) *The Moral Order of Suffering. Plenary Session, Dimensions of Suffering: a Perspective from Palliative Care*. National Conference sponsored by Daw House Hospice and the Flinders, University of South Australia, September 1998.

Clark, D. and Seymour, J. (1999) *Reflections on Palliative Care*. Buckingham: Open University Press.

Clark, P.G. (1995) Quality of life, values and teamwork in geriatric care: do we communicate what we mean?, *Gerontologist*, 35(3): 402–11.

Clark, P.G. (1996) Communication between provider and patient: values, biography, and empowerment in clinical practice, *Ageing and Society*, 16(6): 747–74.

Clarke, C. and Watson, D. (1991) Informal carers of the dementing elderly: a study of relationships, *Nursing Practice*, 4(4): 17–21.

Clarke, D.C. and Fawcett, J. (1992) Review of empirical risk factors for evaluation of the suicidal patient, in B. Bongar (ed.) *Suicide: Guidelines for Assessment, Management and Treatment*. New York: Oxford University Press.

Clarke, T., Abbenbroek, B. and Hardy, L. (1996) The impact of a high dependency unit continuing education program on nursing practice and patient outcomes, *Australian Critical Care*, 9(4): 138–42.

Cleary, J.F. and Carbone, P.P. (1997) Palliative medicine in the elderly, *Cancer*, 80(7): 1335–47.

Clinical Standards Advisory Group (CSAG) (1998) *Community Health Care for Elderly People*. London: HMSO.

Closs, S.J. (1996) Pain and elderly patients: a survey of nurses' knowledge and experiences, *Journal of Advanced Nursing*, 23(2): 237–42.

Cohen, C.A., Pushkar-Gold, D., Shulman, K.I. and Zucchero, C.A. (1994) Positive aspects in Caregiving: an overlooked variable in research, *Canadian Journal of Aging*, 13(3): 378–91.

Cohen-Mansfield, J., Rabinovich, B.A., Lipson, S. *et al.* (1991) The decision to execute a durable power of attorney for health care and preferences regarding the utilization of life sustaining treatments in nursing home residents, *Archives of Internal Medicine*, 151(2): 289–94.

Cohen-Mansfield, J., Marx, M.S. and Werner, P.M. (1992) Agitation in elderly persons: an integrative report of findings in a nursing home, *International Psychogeriatrics*, 4(suppl. 2): 221–40.

Coleman, P. (1997) The last scene of all, *Generations Review*, 7(1): 2–5.

Collins, C.E., Given, B.A. and Given, C.W. (1994) Interventions with family caregivers of persons with Alzheimer's disease, *Nursing Clinics of North America*, 29(1): 195–207.

Conn, V.S. and Armer, J.M. (1996) Gerontological nursing: the time for health promotion (editorial), *Journal of Gerontological Nursing*, December: 5–6.

Connel, C.M. and Gibson, G.D. (1997) Racial, ethnic and cultural differences in dementia caregiving: reviews and analysis, *Gerontologist*, 37(3): 355–64.

Connor, P.A. and Kooker, B.M. (1996) Nurses' knowledge, attitudes, and practices in managing urinary incontinence in the acute care setting, *MEDSURG Nursing*, 5(2): 87–92.

Cookman, C.A. (1996) Older people and attachment to things, places, pets, and ideas, *Image: Journal of Nursing Scholarship*, 28(3): 227–31.

Cooper, S.A. (1997a) Epidemiology of psychiatric disorders in elderly compared with younger adults with learning disabilities, *British Journal of Psychiatry*, 170: 375–80.

Cooper, S.A. (1997b) High prevalence of dementia among people with learning disabilities not attributable to Down's syndrome, *Psychological Medicine*, 27: 609–16.

Cooper, S.A. (1998) Clinical study of the effects of age on the physical health of adults with mental retardation, *American Journal on Mental Retardation*, 102(6): 582–9.

Cooper, S.A. (1999) Learning disabilities and dementia, in J. Keady and S. Cox (eds) *Younger People with Dementia: Planning, Practice and Development*. London: Jessica Kingsley.

Cope, D.N. and Sundance, P. (1995) Conceptualising clinical outcomes, in P.K. Landrum, N.D. Schmidt and A.J. McLean (eds) *Outcome Orientated Rehabilitation: Principles, Strategies and Tools for Effective Program Management*. Gaithersburg, MD: Aspen.

Corbin, J.M. and Strauss, A. (1988) *Unending Work and Care: Managing Chronic Illness at Home*. San Francisco, CA: Jossey Bass.

Corbin, J.M. and Strauss, A. (1991) A nursing model of chronic illness management based upon the trajectory framework, *Scholarly Inquiry for Nursing Practice*, 5(3): 155–74.

Corcoran, M. and Gitlin, L. (1992) Dementia management: an occupational therapy home based intervention for caregivers, *American Journal of Occupational Therapy*, 46(9): 801–8.

Corner, J. and Dunlop, R. (1997) New approaches to care, in D. Clark, J. Hockley and S. Ahmedzai (eds) *New Themes in Palliative Care*. Buckingham: Open University Press.

Costello, J. (1996) Acknowledging loss, *Elderly Care*, 8(4): 35–6.

Cotten, P.D. and Spirrison, C.L. (1991) Mental health needs of the elderly with mental retardation, in M.S. Harper (ed.) *Management and Care of the Elderly: Psychological Perspectives*. London: Sage.

Cotter, A., Meyer., J. and Roberts, S. (1998) Humanity or bureaucracy? The transition from hospital to long-term continuing care, *NT Research*, 3(4): 247–56.

Cox, E.O. and Dooley, A.C. (1996) Care-receivers' perception of their role in the care process, *Journal of Gerontological Social Work*, 26(1/2): 133–52.

Coyle, J. (1999) Exploring the meaning of 'dissatisfaction' with health care: the importance of personal identity threat, *Sociology of Health and Illness*, 21(1): 95–124.

Cruz, V., Abdul Hamid, M. and Heater, B. (1997) Research-based practice: reducing restraints in an acute care setting-phase I, *Journal of Gerontological Nursing*, 23(2): 31–40.

Cuijpers, P. (1998) Psychological outreach programmes for the depressed elderly: a meta-analysis of effects and dropout, *International Journal of Geriatric Psychiatry*, 13(1): 41–8.

Dahlin-lvanoff, S., Klepp, K.I. and Sjostrand, J. (1998) Development of a health education programme for elderly with age related macular degeneration: a focus group study, *Patient Education and Counseling*, 34: 63–73.

Daley, O.E. (1993) Women's strategies for living in a nursing home, *Journal of Gerontological Nursing*, 19(9): 5–9.

Dalley, G. (1998) Health and social welfare policy, in M. Bernard and J. Phillips (eds) *The Social Policy of Old Age: Moving into the 21st Century*. London: Centre for Policy on Ageing.

Dalley, G. (2000) Defining difference: health and social care for older people, in A. Warnes, L. Warren and M. Nolan (eds) *Care Services for Later Life: Transformations and Critiques*. London: Jessica Kingsley.

Daniels, L. (1999) Primary-led palliative care (editorial), *British Journal of Community Care*, 4(3): 108.

Dargie, C., Dawson, S. and Gorside, P. (1999) *Trends in UK Health and implications up until 2015*, Policy future for UK Health, Pathfinder. London: Nuffield Trust.

Davies, B. and O'Berle, K. (1990) Dimensions of the supportive role of the nurse in palliative care, *Oncology Nursing Forum*, 17(1): 87–94.

Davies, C. (1998) Caregiving, carework and professional care, in A. Brechin, J. Walmsley, J. Katz and S. Peace (eds) *Care Matters: Concepts, Practice and Research in Health and Social Care*. London: Sage.

Davies, S. and Nolan, M. (1998) Educating nursing home staff in the reduction of pressure sores, *British Journal of Nursing*, 7(3): 144, 146, 148–51.

Davies, S., Laker, S. and Ellis, L. (1997) Promoting autonomy and independence for older people within nursing practice: a literature review, *Journal of Advanced Nursing*, 26(2): 408–17.

Davies, S., Nolan, M., Brown, J. and Wilson, F. (1999) *Dignity on the Ward: Promoting Excellence in Care*. London: Help the Aged.

Davies, S., Sandberg, J. and Lundh, U. (2000) The entry to a nursing home: residents' and relatives' experiences, in A. Warnes, L. Warren and M. Nolan (eds) *Care Services for Later Life: Transformations and Critiques*. Jessica Kingsley.

Davis, J.A. (1997) 'More than giving out the pills': changing attitudes to aged care through continuing education, *Geriaction*, 15(2): 9–12.

Davis, L.L. (1996) Dementia caregiving studies: a typology for family interventions, *Journal of Family Nursing*, 2(1): 30–55.

Day, H. and Jankey, S.G. (1996) Lessons from the literature: towards a holistic model of quality for life, in R. Renwick, I. Brown and M. Nagler (eds) *Quality of Life in Health Promotion and Rehabilitation: Conceptual Approaches, Issues and Applications*. Thousand Oaks, CA: Sage.

Degner, L. and Gow, C. (1991) Critical nursing behaviors in care for the dying, *Cancer Nursing*, 14(5): 246–53.

Dejong, G. and Sutton, J.P. (1995) Rehabilitation 2000: the evolution of medical rehabilitation in American Health Care, in P.K. Landrum, N.D. Schmidt and A.J. McLean (eds) *Outcome Orientated Rehabilitation: Principles, Strategies and Tools for Effective Program Management*. Gaithersburg, MD: Aspen.

DeLetter, M.C., Tully, C.L., Wilson, J.F. and Rich, E.C. (1995) Nursing staff perceptions of quality of life of cognitively impaired elders: instrumental development, *Journal of Applied Gerontology*, 14(4): 426–43.

Dellasega, C. and Mastrian, K. (1995) The process and consequences of institutionalizing an elder, *Western Journal of Nursing Research*, 17(2): 123–36.

Denney, A. (1997) Quiet dinner music: an intervention for mealtime agitation?, *Journal of Gerontological Nursing*, 23(7): 16–23.

Dent, O.F., Waite, L.M., Bennett, H.P. *et al.* (1999) A longitudinal study of chronic disease and depressive symptoms in a community sample of older people, *Aging and Mental Health*, 3(4): 351–7.

DePaola, S.J. and Ebersole, P. (1995) Meaning in life categories of elderly nursing home residents, *International Journal of Aging and Human Development*, 40(3): 227–36.

Department of Health (1989a) *Caring for People: Community Care in the Next Decade and Beyond*. London: HMSO.

Department of Health (1989b) *Working for Patients*. London: HMSO.

Department of Health (1990) *The NHS and Community Care Act*. London: HMSO.

Department of Health (1991a) *Care Management and Assessment: Summary of Practice Guidance*. London: HMSO.

Department of Health (1991b) *Care Management and Assessment: Practitioners' Guide*. London: HMSO.

Department of Health (1994) *Working in Partnership: a Collaborative Approach to Care*. London: HMSO.

Department of Health (1995a) *Carers (Recognition and Services) Act*. London: HMSO.

Department of Health (1995b) *The Challenge for Nursing and Midwifery in the 21st Century*. Report of the consultation exercise on the 'Heathrow Debate'. London: HMSO.

Department of Health (1995c) *Building Bridges*. London: HMSO.

Department of Health (1996) *Assessing Older People with Dementia in the Community: Practice Issues for Social and Health Services*. Wetherby: HMSO.

Department of Health (1997a) *The New NHS, Modern Dependable*. London: The Stationery Office.

Department of Health (1997b) *A Handbook on the Mental Health of Older People – The Health of the Nations: Mental Illness Key Area.* London: HMSO.

Department of Health (1997c) *At Home with Dementia: Inspection of Services for Older People with Dementia in the Community.* London: HMSO.

Department of Health (1998a) *A First Class Service: Quality in the New NHS.* London: Department of Health.

Department of Health (1998b) *Modernising Social Services: Promoting Independence, Improving Protection, Reviewing Standards.* London: The Stationery Office.

Department of Health (1998c) *Modernising Health and Social Services: National Priorities Guidance 1999–2000–2001–2002.* London: Department of Health.

Department of Health (1999a) *The Carers' National Strategy.* London: The Stationery Office.

Department of Health (1999b) *Our Healthier Nation.* London: The Stationery Office.

Department of Health (1999c) *Making a Difference: Strengthening the Nursing, Midwifery and Health Visiting Contribution to Health and Healthcare.* London: The Stationery Office.

De Raeve, L. (1996) Dignity and integrity at the end of life, *International Journal of Palliative Care Nursing,* 2(2): 71–6.

Devine, A. and Baxter, T.D. (1995) Introducing clinical supervision: a guide, *Nursing Standard,* 9(40): 32–4.

Dhooper, S.S. (1991) Caregivers of Alzheimer's disease patients: a review of the literature, *Journal of Gerontological Social Work,* 18(1): 19–37.

Dodds, P. (1994) Wandering: a short report on coping strategies adopted by informal carers, *International Journal of Geriatric Psychiatry,* 9(9): 751–6.

Donaldson, C., Tarrier, N. *et al.* (1998) Determinants of carer stress in Alzheimer's Disease, *International Journal of Geriatric Psychiatry,* 13(4): 248–56.

Dossa, P.A. (1990) Toward social system theory: implications for older people with developmental disabilities and service delivery, *International Journal of Aging and Human Development,* 30(4): 303–19.

Dowd, T.T. and Campbell, J.M. (1995) Urinary incontinence in an acute care setting, *Journal of Urological Nursing,* 15(3): 82–5.

Downs, M. (1994) *Dementia: a Literature Review for the Northern Ireland Dementia Policy Scrutiny.* Stirling: Dementia Services Development Centre, University of Stirling.

Doyle, C.J. (1995) Effect of staff turnover and the social environment on depressive symptoms in nursing home residents, *International Psychogeriatrics,* 7(1): 51–61.

Dreyfuss, H.L. and Dreyfuss, S.E. (1986) *Mind over Machine: the Power of Human Intuition and Expertise in the Era of the Computer.* Oxford: Basil Blackwell.

Drysdale, A.E., Nelson, C.F. and Wineman, N.M. (1993) Families need help too: group treatment for families of nursing home residents, *Clinical Nurse Specialist,* 7(3): 130–4.

Dunst, C.J., Trivette, C.M., Starnes, A.L., Hamby, D.W. and Gordon, N.J. (1993) *Building and Evaluating Family Support Initiatives.* Baltimore, MD: Paul H. Brookes.

Dunst, C.J., Trivette, C.M. and Deal, A.G. (1994) *Supporting and Strengthening Families: Volume 1, Methods, Strategies and Practices.* Cambridge, MA: Brookline.

Dunstan, E. (1996) '. . . and a time to die': the medicine of old age, *British Medical Bulletin,* 52(2): 255–62.

Easterbrook, L. (1999) *When We are Very Old: Reflections on Treatment Care and Support of Older People.* London: King's Fund.

Ebrahim, S. (1994) The goals of rehabilitation for older people, *Reviews in Clinical Gerontology*, 4(2): 93–6.

Ebrahim, S., Wallis, C., Brittis, S., Harwood, R. and Graham, N. (1993) Long term care for elderly people, *Quality in Health Care*, 2: 198–203.

Edgerton, R.B. (1967) *The Cloak of Competence: Stigma in the Lives of the Mentally Retarded*. Berkeley, CA: University of California Press.

Edgerton, R.B. and Gaston, M.A. (1991) *'I've Seen It All': Lives of Older Persons with Mental Retardation in the Community*. Baltimore, MD: Paul H. Brookes.

Edgerton, R.B., Bollinger, M. and Herr, B. (1984) The cloak of competence: after two decades, *American Journal of Mental Deficiency*, 88: 345–51.

Edgerton, R.B., Gaston, M.A., Kelly, H. and Ward, T.W. (1994) Health care for ageing people with mental retardation, *Mental Retardation*, 32(2): 146–50.

Eraut, M. (1994) *Developing Professional Knowledge and Competence*. London: Falmer.

Erickson, M., Krauss, M.W. and Seltzer, M.M. (1989) Perceptions of old age among a sample of ageing mentally retarded persons, *Journal of Applied Gerontology*, 8(2): 251–60.

Espino, D. and Bradley, A.J. (1998) Diagnostic approach to the confused elderly patient, *American Family Physician*, 57(6): 1358–66.

Espino, D. and Lewis, R. (1998) Dementia in older minority populations – issues of prevalence, diagnosis and treatment, *American Journal of Geriatric Psychiatry*, 6(2): 519–25.

Evandrou, M. (1998) Great expectations: social policy and the new millennium elders, in M. Bernard and J. Phillips (eds) *The Social Policy of Old Age: Moving into the 21st Century*. London: Centre for Policy on Ageing.

Evans, G. (1994) Supporting role . . . independent advocates can enhance communication between the professionals and the older people they are caring for, *Nursing Times*, 90(9): 70–1.

Evans, J. (1997) The clinical achievements of British geriatrics, in J. Phillips (ed.) *British Gerontology and Experience and Innovation*. British Geriatric Society, British Society for Research on Ageing and British Society of Gerontology.

Evans, L.K. (1996) Knowing the patient: the route to individualized care, *Journal of Gerontological Nursing*, 22(3): 15–19.

Evans, M. (1999) *Ethics: Reconciling Conflicting Values in Health Policy*, Policy Futures for UK Health no. 9. London: Nuffield Trust.

Evans, R.L., Connis, R.T., Hendricks, R.D. and Haselkorn, J.K. (1995) Multidisciplinary rehabilitation versus medical care: a meta-analysis, *Social Science and Medicine*, 40(12): 1699–706.

Evenhuis, H.M. (1995) Medical aspects of ageing in a population with intellectual disability: 1. visual impairment, *Journal of Intellectual Disability Research*, 39(1): 18–25.

Evenhuis, H.M., Henderson, C.M., Beange, H., Lennox, N. and Chicoine, B. (2000) *Healthy Ageing – Adults with Intellectual Disabilities: Physical Health Issues*. Geneva: World Health Organisation.

Evers, H.K. (1991) Care of the elderly sick in the UK, in S.J. Redfern (ed.) *Nursing Elderly People*. Edinburgh: Churchill Livingstone.

Exton-Smith, A.N. (1961) Terminal illness in the aged, *Lancet*, 2: 305–8.

Fagermoen, M.S. (1997) Professional identity: values embedded in meaningful nursing practice, *Journal of Advanced Nursing*, 25(3): 434–41.

Farrell, C., Robinson, J. and Fletcher, P. (1999) *A New Era for Community Care? What People Want from Health, Housing and Social Care Agencies*. London: King's Fund.

Farquhar, M. (1995) Elderly people's definitions of quality of life, *Social Science and Medicine*, 41(10): 1439–46.

Faux, S.A. and Seideman, R.Y. (1996) Health care professionals and their relationships with families who have members with developmental disabilities, *Journal of Family Nursing*, 2(7): 217–38.

Felce, D. and Perry, J. (1996) Exploring current conceptions of quality of life: a model for people with and without disabilities, in R. Renwick, I. Brown, and M. Nagler (eds) *Quality of Life in Health Promotion and Rehabilitation*. Thousand Oaks, CA: Sage.

Felce, D., Grant, G., Todd, S. *et al.* (1998) *Towards a Full Life: Researching Policy Innovation for People with Learning Disabilities*. Oxford: Butterworth Heinemann.

Feldman, S. (1999) Please don't call me 'dear': older women's narratives of health, *Nursing Inquiry*, 6: 269–76.

Ferrell, B.A. (1995) Pain evaluation and management in the nursing home. *Annals of Internal Medicine*, 123(9): 681–7.

Ferrell, B.A. and Ferrell, B.R. (1993) Pain assessment among cognitively impaired nursing home residents, *Journal of the American Geriatrics Society*, 41(4): 24–7.

Field, D. (1994) Palliative medicine and the medicalization of death, *European Journal of Cancer Care*, 3: 58–62.

Fife, B.L. (1995) The measurement of meaning in illness, *Social Science and Medicine*, 40(8): 1021–8.

Fitting, M., Rabins, P., Lucas, M.J. and Eastham, J. (1986) Caregivers for dementia patients: a comparison of husbands and wives, *Gerontologist*, 26(3): 248–59.

Fitzgerald, J. (1998) *Time for Freedom? Services for Older People with Learning Difficulties*. London: Joseph Rowntree Foundation, Centre for Policy on Ageing, Values into Action.

Fitzgerald, M. (1999) The experience of chronic illness: a phenomological approach, in R. Nay and S. Garrat (eds) *Nursing Older People: Issues and Innovations*. Sydney: Maclennan and Petty.

Fitzpatrick, R. (1996) Patient centred approaches to the evaluation of health care, in K.W.M. Fulford, S. Ersser and T. Hope (eds) *Essential Practice in Patient Centred Care*. Oxford: Blackwell Science.

Foelker, G.A. and Luke, E.A. (1989) Mental health issues for the aging mentally retarded population, *Journal of Applied Gerontology*, 8: 242–50.

Folkman, S. (1997) Positive psychological states and coping with severe stress, *Social Science and Medicine*, 45: 1207–21.

Fontana, J.A. (1995) A consideration of vigor as an outcome measure of exercise therapy in chronic illness, *Rehabilitation Nursing Research*, 4(3): 75–81.

Ford, K., Middleton, J., Palmer, B. and Farrington, A. (1997) Primary healthcare workers: training needs in mental health, *British Journal of Nursing*, 6(21): 1244–50.

Ford, P. and Keady, J. (1997) Assessment of older people with mental health needs, *Elderly Care*, 9(2): 12–14, 16–17.

Ford, P. and McCormack, B. (1999) The key attributes of a gerontological nurse specialist, *Nursing Standard*, 13(33): 31.

Forrest, J. (1995) Assessment of acute and chronic pain in older adults, *Journal of Gerontological Nursing*, 21(10): 15–20.

Fossbinder, D. (1994) Patient perceptions of nursing care, *Journal of Advanced Nursing*, 20: 1085–93.

Francis, D., Fletcher, K. and Simon, L.J. (1998) The geriatric resource nurse model of care, *Nursing Clinics of North America*, 33(3): 481–98.

Frenn, M. (1996) Older adults' experience of health promotion: a theory for nursing practice, *Public Health Nursing*, 13(1): 65–71.

Fruin, D. (1998) *A Matter of Chance for Carers? Inspection of Local Authority Support for Carers*. Wetherby: Social Services Inspectorate/Department of Health.

Fulmer, T. and Abraham, I.L. (1998) Rethinking geriatric nursing, *Nursing Clinics of North America*, 33(3): 387–94.

Gallagher, S. and Mechanic, D. (1996) Living with the mentally ill: effects on the health and functioning of other household members, *Social Science and Medicine*, 42(12): 1691–701.

Gamble, E.R., McDonald, P.J. and Lichstein, P.R. (1991) Knowledge, attitudes, and behaviour of elderly people regarding living wills, *Archives of Internal Medicine*, 151(2): 277–80.

Gammon, C. (1995) Palliative care for all?, *British Medical Journal*, 1410: 310.

Garwick, A.W., Detzner, D. and Boss, P. (1994) Family perceptions of living with Alzheimer's disease, *Family Process*, 33(3): 327–40.

George, R. and Sykes, J. (1997) Beyond cancer?, in D. Clark, J. Hockley and S. Ahmedzai (eds) *New Themes in Palliative Care*. Buckingham: Open University Press.

Gerhardt, U. (1990) Qualitative research on chronic illness – the issue and the story, *Social Science and Medicine*, 30(11): 1149–59.

Gibb, H. and O'Brien, B. (1990) Jokes and reassurance are not enough: ways in which nurses relate through conversations with elderly clients, *Journal of Advanced Nursing*, 15: 1389–401.

Gibbs, G. (1995) Nurses in private nursing homes: a study of their knowledge and attitudes to pain management in palliative care, *Palliative Medicine*, 9: 245–53.

Gillick, M.R. and Mendes, M.L. (1996) Medical care in old age: what do nurses in long-term care consider appropriate?, *Journal of the American Geriatric Society*, 44(11): 1322–5.

Gillis, K.J. and Hirdes, J.P. (1996) The quality of life implications of health practices among older adults: evidence from the 1991 Canadian General Social Survey, *Canadian Journal on Aging*, 15(2): 299–314.

Gilloran, A., McGlew, T., McKee, K., Robertson, A. and Wight, D. (1994) Measuring the quality of care in psychogeriatric wards, *Journal of Advanced Nursing*, 18: 269–75.

Given, B.A. and Given, C.W. (1991) Family caregivers for the elderly, in J. Fitzpatrick, R. Tauton and A. Jacox (eds) *Annual Review of Nursing Research*, vol. 9. New York: Springer.

Gladstone, J.W. (1995) The marital perceptions of elderly persons living or having a spouse living in a long-term care institution in Canada, *Gerontologist*, 35(1): 52–60.

Glass, T.A., Kasl, S.V. and Berkman, L.F. (1997) Stressful life events and depressive symptoms among the elderly: evidence from a prospective community study, *Journal of Aging and Mental Health*, 9(1): 70–89.

Gluck, T., Wientjes, H.J. and Rai, G.S. (1996) An evaluation of risk factors for inpatient falls in acute and rehabilitation elderly care wards, *Gerontology*, 42(2): 104–7.

Glueckauf, R.L., Sechrest, L.B., Bord, G.R. and McDonel, E.G. (eds) (1993) *Improving Assessment in Rehabilitation and Health*. Newbury Park, CA: Sage.

Glyn-Hughes, H.L. (1960) *Peace at Last.* London: Calouste Gulbenkian Foundation.

Goldsmith, M. (1996) *Hearing the Voice of People with Dementia: Opportunities and Obstacles.* London: Jessica Kingsley.

Gonzales, E., Gitlin, L.N. and Lyons, K.J. (1995) Review of the literature on African American care caregivers of individuals with dementia, *Journal of Cultural Diversity*, 2(2): 40–8.

Goodwinjohansson, C. (1996) How caregivers can affect quality of life in the nursing home, *Topics in Geriatric Rehabilitation*, 11(4): 25–33.

Gournay, K. (1994) Redirecting the emphasis to serious mental illness, *Nursing Times*, 90(25): 40–1.

Graham, H. and Livesley, B. (1983) Dying as diagnosis: difficulties of communication and management in elderly patients, *Lancet,* 13 September: 670–2.

Graham, I.W. (1999) Reflective narrative and dementia care, *Journal of Clinical Nursing*, 8(6): 675–83.

Grainger, C.V., Kelly-Hayes, M., Johnston, M. *et al.* (1996) Quality and outcome measures for medical rehabilitation, in R.M. Buschbacker, D. Dumitru, E.W. Johnson, D. Matthews and M. Sinahe (eds) *Physical Medicine and Rehabilitation.* Philadelphia, PA: Saunders.

Grainger, K. (1993) That's a lovely bath dear: reality construction in the discourse of elderly care, *Journal of Aging Studies*, 7(3): 247–62.

Grande, G.E., Addington-Hall, J.M. and Todd, C.J. (1998) Place of death and access to home care services: are certain groups at a disadvantage?, *Social Science and Medicine*, 47(5): 565–79.

Grant, G. (1989) Letting go: decision-making among family carers of people with a mental handicap, *Australia and New Zealand Journal of Developmental Disabilities*, 15(3/4): 189–200.

Grant, G. (1990) Elderly parents with handicapped children: anticipating the future, *Journal of Ageing Studies*, 4(4): 359–74.

Grant, G. and Ramcharan, P. (1999) *Views and Experiences of Users and Carers: a Research Review.* Report for the Department of Health Learning Disability Research Initiative. Sheffield: School of Nursing and Midwifery, University of Sheffield.

Grant, G. and Whittell, B. (1999) *Family Care of People with Learning Disabilities: Support for Family Coping. Final Report to NHS Wales Office of Research and Development.* School of Nursing and Midwifery, University of Sheffield and CSPRD, University of Wales Bangor.

Grant, G., McGrath, M. and Ramcharan, P. (1995) Community inclusion of older people with learning disabilities, *Care in Place: International Journal of Networks and Community*, 2(1): 29–44.

Grant, G., Ramcharan, P., McGrath, M., Nolan, M. and Keady, J. (1998) Rewards and gratification among family caregivers: towards a more refined model of caring and coping, *Journal of Intellectual Disability Research*, 42(1): 58–71.

Grau, L., Chandler, B. and Saunders, C. (1995) Nursing home residents' perceptions of the quality of their care, *Journal of Psychosocial Nursing and Mental Health Services*, 33(5): 34–43.

Greengross, S., Murphy, E., Quam, L., Rochon, P. and Smith, R. (1997) Aging: a subject that must be at the top of the world agendas, *British Medical Journal*, 315: 1029–30.

Gregory, D. and English, J. (1996) The myth of control: suffering in palliative care, *Journal of Palliative Care*, 10(2): 18–22.

Griffin, F. (1997) Discovering knowledge in practice settings, in S.E. Thorne and V.E. Hayes (eds) *Nursing Praxis: Knowledge and Action*. Thousand Oaks, CA: Sage.

Griffiths, R. (1988*) Community Care: an Agenda for Action*. London: HMSO.

Guarnaccia, P. and Parra, P. (1996) Ethnicity, social status, and families' experiences of caring for a mentally ill family member, *Community Mental Health Journal*, 32(3): 243–60.

Guilmette, T. and Snow, M. (1992) Emotional dysfunction in a geriatric population: staff observations and patients' reports, *Archives of Physical Medicine and Rehabilitation*, 73(6): 587–93.

Gunter, L.M. (1983) Ethical considerations of nursing care of older patients in the acute care setting, *Nursing Clinics of North America*, 18(2): 411–21.

Guthrie, S. and Harvey, A. (1994) Motivation and its influence on outcomes in rehabilitation, *Reviews in Clinical Gerontology*, 4: 235–43.

Haap, M.B., Williams, C.C., Strumpf, N.E. and Burger, S.G. (1996) Individualized care for frail elders: theory and practice, *Journal of Gerontological Nursing*, 22(3): 6–14.

Haas, B.K. (1999) Clarification and integration of similar quality of life concepts, *Image: Journal of Nursing Scholarship*, 31(3): 215–20.

Hall, B.L. and Bocksnick, J.G. (1995) Therapeutic recreation for the institutionalized elderly: choice or abuse, *Journal of Elder Abuse and Neglect*, 7(4): 49–60.

Halldorsdottir, S. (1997) Implications of the caring/competence dichotomy, in S.E. Thorne and V.E. Jaues (eds) *Nursing Praxis: Knowledge and Action*. Thousand Oaks, CA: Sage.

Hamid, W. and Silverman, M. (1995) Needs assessment in old-age psychiatry: a need for standardization, *International Journal of Geriatric Psychiatry*, 10(7): 533–40.

Hamilton, L. and Lyon, P.S. (1995) A nursing-driven program to preserve and restore functional ability in hospitalized elderly patients, *Journal of Nursing Administration*, 25(4): 30–7.

Hancock, R., Bender, P., Dayhoff, N. and Nyhuis, A. (1996) Factors associated with nursing interventions to reduce incontinence in hospitalized older adults, *Journal of Urological Nursing*, 16(3): 79–85.

Hand, J.E. (1994) Report of a national survey of older people with lifelong intellectual handicap in New Zealand, *Journal of Intellectual Disability Research*, 38: 275–87.

Hanestad, B.R. (1996) Nurses' perceptions of the content, relevance and usefulness of the quality of life concept in relation to nursing practice [corrected] [published erratum appears in *Vard I Norden*, 1996; 16(2): 33], *Vard I Norden Nursing Science and Research in the Nordic Countries*, 16(1): 17–21.

Hanford, L., Easterbrook, L. and Stevenson, J. (1999) *Rehabilitation for Older People: The Emerging Policy Agenda*. London: King's Fund.

Hanrahan, P. and Luchins, D. (1995) Access to hospice programs in end-stage dementia: a national survey of hospice programs, *Journal of the American Geriatric Society*, 43: 56–9.

Hanson, E. and Culihall, K. (1995) Images of palliative nursing care, *Journal of Palliative Care*, 11(3): 35–9.

Hanson, E.S. and Clarke, A. (2000) The role of telematics in assisting family carers and frail older people at home, *Health and Social Care in the Community*, 8(2): 232–41.

Hanson, E.S., Tetley, J. and Clarke, A. (2000) A multimedia intervention to support family carers. *Gerontologist*, 39(6): 736–41.

Harber, D. (1989) *Health Care for an Aging Society.* New York: Hemisphere.

Hardman, C.S., Guy, P.M., Dunn, R.B., Lewis, P.A. and Vetter, N.J. (1995) Health visiting elderly people after discharge from hospital, *Health Visitor*, 68(9): 370–1.

Hardy, B., Young, R. and Wistow, G. (1999) Dimensions of choice in the assessment and care management process: the views of older people, carers and care managers, *Health and Social Care in the Community*, 7(6): 483–91.

Harper, D.C. and Wadsworth, J.S. (1990) Dementia and depression in elders with mental retardation: a pilot study, *Research in Developmental Disabilities*, 11: 177–98.

Harper, S. (2000) Ageing 2000: questions for the twenty first century, *Ageing and Society*, 20(1): 111–22.

Harris, L. (1990) The disadvantaged dying, *Nursing Times*, 86(22): 26–9.

Harris, P.B. (1993) The misunderstood caregiver? A qualitative study of the male caregiver of Alzheimer's disease victims, *Gerontologist*, 33: 551–6.

Harvath, T.A. (1994) Interpretation and management of dementia-related behaviour problems, *Clinical Nursing Research*, 3(1): 7–26.

Harvath, T.A., Archbold, P.G., Stewart, B.J. *et al.* (1994) Establishing partnerships with family caregivers: local and cosmopolitan knowledge, *Journal of Gerontological Nursing*, 20(2): 29–35.

Hasselkus, B.R. (1994) From hospital to home: family–professional relationships in geriatric rehabilitation, *Gerontology and Geriatrics Education*, 15(1): 91–100.

Hasselkus, B.R., Dickie, V.A. and Gregory, C. (1997) Geriatric occupational therapy: the uncertain ideology of long-term care, *American Journal of Occupational Therapy*, 51(2): 132–9.

Haveman, M., Maaskant, M.A. and Sturmans, F. (1989) Older Dutch residents of institutions, with and without Down syndrome: comparison of mortality and morbidity trends and motor/social functioning, *Australia and New Zealand Journal of Developmental Disabilities*, 15: 241–55.

Hawley, D. and DeHaan, L. (1996) Towards a definition of family resilience: integrating lifespan and family perspectives, *Family Process*, 35: 283–98.

Health Advisory Service (1982) *The Rising Tide.* Sutton, Surrey: National Health Service.

Health Advisory Service (1997) *Services for People who are Elderly: Addressing the Balance.* London: The Stationery Office.

Health Advisory Service (HAS) 2000 (1998) *'Not Because They are Old': an Independent Inquiry into the Care of Older People on Acute Wards in General Hospitals.* London: Health Advisory Service 2000.

Health Advisory Service (HAS) 2000 (1999) *Standards for Mental Health Services for Older People.* Brighton: Pavilion.

Health Education Authority (1998) *Older People in the Population, Fact Sheet 1.* London: The Stationery Office.

Heap, M.J., Munglani, R., Klinck, J.R. and Males, A.G. (1993) Elderly patients' preferences concerning life-support treatment, *Anaesthesia*, 48(120): 1027–33.

Heath, H. and Ford, P. (1996) *Older People and Nursing: Issues of Living in a Care Home.* Oxford: Butterworth Heinemann.

Heintz, A.P.M. (1994) Euthanasia: can be part of good terminal care, *British Medical Journal*, 308: 1656.

Hektor, L.M. and Touhy, T.A. (1997) The history of the bath: from art to task? Reflections for the future, *Journal of Gerontological Nursing*, 23(5): 7–15.

Heller, A. and Factor, A. (1993) Support systems, well-being, and placement decision-making among older parents and their adult children with developmental disabilities, in E. Sutton, A. Factor, B.A. Hawkins, A. Heller and G.B. Seltzer (eds) *Older Adults with Developmental Disabilities: Optimizing Choice and Change*. Baltimore, MD: Paul H. Brookes.

Heller, T. (1993) Ageing caregivers of persons with developmental disabilities: changes in burden and placement desire, in K.A. Roberto (ed.) *The Elderly Caregiver: Caring for Adults with Developmental Disabilities*. Newbury Park, CA: Sage.

Heller, T. and Roccoforte, J. (1997) Predictors of support group participation among families of persons with mental illness, *Family Relations*, 46(4): 437–42.

Henderson, J.A. and Vesperi, M.D. (1995) *The Culture of Long Term Care: Nursing Home Ethnography*. New York: Bergin and Garvey.

Henwood, M. (1992) *Through a Glass Darkly: Community Care and Elderly People*. London: King's Fund Institute.

Henwood, M. (1998) *Ignored and Invisible? Carers' Experience of the NHS*. Report of a UK research survey commissioned by Carers' National Association.

Herbert, G. (1997) *Sharing the Caring: Learning Together – A Joint Review of Services for Older People with Mental Health Problems in North Yorkshire and the City of York*. Leeds: Nuffield Institute for Health, University of Leeds.

Herring, R. and Thom, B. (1997) Alcohol misuse in older people: the role of home carers, *Health and Social Care in the Community*, 5(4): 237–45.

Hershenson, D.B. (1990) A theoretical model for rehabilitation counselling, *Rehabilitation Counselling Bulletin*, 33(4): 268–78.

Herzberg, S.R. (1993) Positioning the nursing home resident: an issue of quality of life, *American Journal of Occupational Therapy*, 47(1): 75–7.

Higginson, I. (1993) Palliative care: a review of past changes and future trends, *Journal of Public Health Medicine*, 15: 3–8.

Hinton, J. (1979) Comparison of places and policies for terminal care, *Lancet*, 6 January: 29–32.

Hirschfield, M.J. (1981) Families living and coping with the cognitively impaired, in L.A. Copp (ed.) *Care of the Ageing: Recent Advances in Nursing*. Edinburgh: Churchill Livingstone.

Hirschfield, M.J. (1983) Home care versus institutionalization: family caregiving and senile brain disease, *International Journal of Nursing Studies*, 20(1): 23–32.

Hoeman, S.P. (1996) Conceptual bases for rehabilitation nursing, in S.P. Hoeman (ed.) *Rehabilitation Nursing: Process and Application*. St Louis, MO: Mosby.

Hofman, A., Rocca, W.A., Brayne, C. *et al.* (1991) The prevalence of dementia in Europe: a collaborative study in 1980–1990 findings, *International Journal of Epidemiology*, 20(3): 736–48.

Hogg, J. and Lambe, L. (1998) *Older People with Learning Disabilities: a Review of the Literature on Residential Services and Family Caregiving*. London: Foundation for People with Learning Disabilities.

Hogg, J. and Moss, S. (1993) Characteristics of older people with intellectual disabilities in England, in N.W. Bray (ed.) *International Review of Research in Mental Retardation*, vol. 19. London: Academic Press.

Hogg, J., Lucchino, R., Wang, K. and Janicki, M. and working group (2000) *Healthy Ageing – Adults with Intellectual Disabilities: Ageing and Social Policy*. Geneva: World Health Organisation.

Hogstel, M.O. and Cox, M. (1995) Hospital resources for care of acutely ill older persons, *Journal of Gerontological Nursing*, 21(11): 25–31.

House of Commons Health Committee (1996) *Review of Long-term Care*. London: HMSO.

Howarth, G. (1998) 'Just live for today': living, caring, ageing and dying, *Ageing and Society*, 18: 673–89.

Howse, K. (1998) Health care rationing, non-treatment and euthanasia: ethical dilemmas, in M. Bernard and J. Phillips (eds) *The Social Policy of Old Age: Moving into the 21st Century*. London: Centre for Policy on Ageing.

Hudson, K.A. and Sexton, D.L. (1996) Perceptions about nursing care: comparing elders' and nurses' priorities, *Journal of Gerontological Nursing*, 22(12): 41–6.

Hughes, B. (1995) *Older People and Community Care: Critical Theory and Practice*. Buckingham: Open University Press.

Hunt, T.E. (1980) Practical considerations in the rehabilitation of the aged, *Journal of the American Geriatrics Society*, 28: 59–64.

Hutton, J. (1999) Address to Dignity on the Ward Conference, London: November 1999. *Conference Proceedings*. London: Help the Aged.

Hymovich, D.P. and Hagopian, G.A. (1992) *Chronic Illness in Children and Adults: a Psychosocial Approach*. Philadelphia, PA: Saunders.

Ide, B.A. and Wolff, T.L. (1993) Vulnerable issues related to rural elder's and non elder's perceptions of community, *Behaviour, Health and Aging*, 3(1): 3–12.

Iliffe, S. (1994) Why GPs have a bad reputation, *Journal of Dementia Care*, 2(6): 24–5.

Impallomeni, M. and Starr, J. (1995) The changing face of community and institutional care for the elderly, *Journal of Public Health Medicine*, 17(2): 171–8.

Ingvad, B. and Olsson, E. (1999) The care relationship as a dynamic aspect of the quality of the home care services. Paper presented at Fourth European Congress of Gerontology, Berlin.

International Association for the Scientific Study of Intellectual Disabilities and Inclusion International (2000) *Ageing and Intellectual Disabilities: Improving Longevity and Promoting Health Ageing*. Summative Report. Geneva: World Health Organisation.

International Association of Gerontology (1998) Adelaide Declaration on Ageing, *Australasian Journal on Ageing*, 17(1): 3–4.

Irurito, V.F. (1996) Hidden dimensions revealed: progressive grounded theory study of quality in hospital care, *Qualitiative Health Research*, 6(3): 331–49.

Iwasiw, C., Goldenberg, D., MacMaster, E., McCutcheon, S. and Bol, N. (1996) Residents' perceptions of their first 2 weeks in a long-term care facility, *Journal of Clinical Nursing*, 5(6): 381–8.

Jacelon, C.S. (1995) The effect of living in a nursing home on socialization in elderly people, *Journal of Advanced Nursing*, 22(3): 539–46.

James, V. and Field, D. (1996) Who has the power? Some problems and issues affecting the nursing care of dying patients, *European Journal of Cancer Care*, 5: 73–80.

Jamieson, S. (1999) HIV-related brain impairment, in S. Cox and J. Keady (eds) *Younger People with Dementia: Planning, Practice and Development*. London: Jessica Kingsley.

Janes, J. (1993) Safe as houses, *Nursing Times*, 89(14): 46–7.

Janes, N.M., Wells, D.L. and Daly, J. (1997) Elderly patients' experiences with nurses guided by Parse's theory of human becoming . . . including commentary by Daly, J., *Clinical Nursing Research*, 6(3): 205–24.

Janicki, M.P. and Jacobson, J.W. (1986) Generational trends in sensory, physical and behavioral abilities among older mentally retarded persons, *American Journal of Mental Deficiency*, 90(5): 490–500.

Janicki, M.P. and MacEachron, A.E. (1984) Residential, health and social service needs of elderly developmentally disabled persons, *Gerontologist*, 24(2): 128–37.

Janicki, M.P., Dalton, A.J., Henderson, C.M. and Davidson, P.W. (1999) Mortality and morbidity among older adults with intellectual disability: health services considerations, *Disability and Rehabilitation*, 21: 284–94.

Jansson, W., Almberg, B. *et al.* (1998) The circle mode: support for relatives of people with dementia, *International Journal of Geriatric Psychiatry*, 13: 674–81.

Jenkins, M., Hildreth, B.L. and Hildreth, G. (1993) Elderly persons with mental retardation: an exceptional population with special needs, *International Journal of Ageing and Human Development*, 37(1): 69–80.

Jensen, L.A. and Allen, M.N. (1994) A synthesis of qualitative research on wellness – illness, *Qualitative Health Research*, 4(4): 349–69.

Johnson, C.L. and Barer, B.M. (1997) *Life beyond 85 Years: the Aura of Survivorship*. New York: Springer.

Johnson, M. (1990) Nursing home placement: the daughter's perspective, *Journal of Gerontological Nursing*, 16(11): 6–11.

Johnson, S., Ramsey, R., Thornicroft, G. *et al.* (1997) *London's Mental Health*. Report for the King's Fund London Commission. London: King's Fund.

Jones, G. and Miesen, B. (1992) *Care-Giving in Dementia: Research and Applications*. London: Routledge.

Jones, J., Dagnan, D., Trower, P. and Ruddick, L. (1996) Persons with learning disabilities living in community-based homes: the relationship of quality of life with age and disability, *International Journal of Rehabilitation Research*, 19: 219–27.

Jordan, F.M., Worrall, L.E., Hickson, L.M. and Dodd, B.J. (1993) The evaluation of intervention programmes for communicatively impaired elderly people, *European Journal of Disorders in Communication*, 28(1): 63–85.

Jorm, A.F., Henderson, A.S., Scott, R. *et al.* (1995) Factors associated with the wish to die in elderly people, *Age and Ageing*, 245: 389–92.

Joseph Rowntree Foundation (1999) *Developing a Preventive Approach with Older People*. York: Joseph Rowntree Foundation.

Kahana, E. and Young, R. (1990) Clarifying the caregiving paradigm: challenges for the future, in D.E. Biegel and A. Blum (eds) *Ageing and Caregiving: Theory, Research and Policy*. Thousand Oaks, CA: Sage.

Kane, R.A. (1999) Goals of home care: therapeutic, compensatory, either or both?, *Journal of Aging and Health*, 11(3): 299–321.

Kane, R., Kane, R., Illston, L., Nyman, J. and Finch, M. (1991) Adult foster-care for the elderly in Oregon – a mainstream alternative to nursing-homes, *American Journal of Public Health*, 81(9): 1113–20.

Kaplan, G.A., Haan, M.N. and Syme, S.L. (1987) Socio-economic position and health, *American Journal of Preventative Medicine*, 3: 125–9.

Kart, C.S. and Dunkle, R.E. (1989) Assessing capacity for self care among the aged, *Journal of Health*, 1: 185–93.

Katz, J., Komaromy, C. and Siddell, M. (1999) Understanding palliative care in residential and nursing homes, *International Journal of Palliative Care Nursing*, 5(2): 58–64.

Kayser Jones, J. (1996) Mealtime in nursing homes: the importance of individualized care, *Journal of Gerontological Nursing*, 22(3): 26–31.

Keady, J. (1996) The experience of dementia: a review of the literature and implications for nursing practice, *Journal of Clinical Nursing*, 5(5): 275–88.

Keady, J. (1999) The dynamics of dementia: a modified grounded theory study. PhD thesis, University of Wales, Bangor.

Keady, J. and Nolan, M. (1996) Behavioural and instrumental stressers in dementia (BISID): refocusing the assessment of caregiver need in dementia, *Journal of Psychiatric and Mental Health Nursing*, 3(3): 163–72.

Keir, D. (1996) Rehabilitation: complex values of a limitless team, in A.J. Squires (ed.) *Rehabilitation of Older People: a Handbook for the MDT.* London: Chapman Hall.

Keith, R.A. (1995) Conceptual basis of outcome measures, *American Journal of Physical Medicine and Rehabilitation*, 77: 73–80.

Keith, R.A. and Lipsey, M.W. (1993) The role of theory in rehabilitation assessment treatment and outcomes, in R.L. Glueckauf, L.B. Sechrest, G.R. Bond and E.G. McDonel (eds) *Improving Assessment in Rehabilitation and Health*. Newbury Park, CA: Sage.

Kellogg, F.R., Crain, M., Corwin, J. and Brickner, P.W. (1992) Life-sustaining interventions in frail elderly persons: talking about choices, *Archives of Internal Medicine*, 152: 2317–20.

Kelly, L.E., Knox, V.J. and Gekoski, W.L. (1998) Women's views of institutional versus community-based long-term care, *Research on Ageing*, 20(2): 218–45.

Kelner, M. (1995) Activists and delegators: elderly patients' preferences about control at the end of life, *Social Science and Medicine*, 41: 537–45.

Kemp, B.J. (1993) Psychological care of older rehabilitation patients, *Clinics in Geriatric Medicine*, 9(4): 841–57.

Kendig, H. and Brooke, C. (1999) Social perspectives on community nursing, in R. Nay and S. Garrat (eds) *Nursing Older People: Issues and Innovations*. Sydney: Maclennan and Petty.

Keown, J. (1995) Euthanasia in the Netherlands: sliding down the slippery slope?, in J. Keown (ed.) *Euthanasia Examined: Ethical, Clinical and Legal Perspectives*. Cambridge: Cambridge University Press.

Kerr, M., Dunstan, F. and Thapar, A. (1996) Attitudes of general practitioners to caring for people with learning disability, *British Journal of General Practice*, 46: 92–4.

Khaw, K-T. (1997) Healthy ageing, *British Medical Journal*, 315: 1090–6.

King's Fund Centre (1984) *Living Well into Old Age: Applying Principles of Good Practice to Services for People with Dementia*, Report no. 63. London: King's Fund.

Kitwood, T. (1988) The technical, the personal and the framing of dementia, *Social Behaviour*, 3: 161–80.

Kitwood, T. (1989) Brain, mind and dementia: with particular reference to Alzheimer's disease, *Ageing and Society*, 9: 1–15.

Kitwood, T. (1990a) Understanding senile dementia: a psychobiographical approach, *Free Associations*, 19: 60–76.

Kitwood, T. (1990b) The dialectics of dementia: with particular reference to Alzheimer's disease, *Ageing and Society*, 10(2): 177–96.

Kitwood, T. (1992) Quality assurance in dementia care, *Geriatric Medicine*, 22(9): 34–8.

Kitwood, T. (1993) Person and process in dementia (editorial), *International Journal of Geriatric Psychiatry*, 8: 541–5.

Kitwood, T. (1997) *Dementia Reconsidered: the Person Comes First*. Buckingham: Open University Press.

Kitwood, T. and Bredin, M. (1992a) Towards a theory of dementia care: personhood and well-being, *Ageing and Society*, 12: 269–87.

Kitwood, T. and Bredin, K. (1992b) A new approach to the evaluation of dementia care, *Journal of Advances in Health and Nursing Care*, 1(5): 41–60.

Kivnick, H.Q. and Murray, S.U. (1997) Vital involvement: an overlooked source of identity in frail elders, *Journal of Aging and Identity*, 2(3): 205–25.

Kleinmann, A. (1995) The social course of chronic illness: delegitimation, resistance and transformation in North American and Chinese societies, in S.K. Toombs, D. Darnard and R.A. Carson (eds) *Chronic Illness: from Experience to Policy.* Bloomington, IN: Indiana University Press.

Kobayashi, S., Masaki, H. and Noguchi, M. (1993) Developmental process: family caregivers of demented Japanese, *Journal of Gerontological Nursing*, 19(10): 7–12.

Koch, T. and Webb, C. (1996) The biomedical construction of ageing: implications for nursing care of older people, *Journal of Advanced Nursing*, 23(5): 954–9.

Koder, D.A., Broadaty, H. and Anstey, K.J. (1996) Cognitive therapy for depression in the elderly, *International Journal of Geriatric Psychiatry*, 11(2): 97–107.

Kovach, S. and Robinson, J. (1996) The roommate relationship for the elderly nursing-home resident, *Journal of Social and Personal Relationships*, 13(4): 627–34.

Kramer, B. (1994) Expanding the conceptualization of caregiver coping – the importance of relationship-focused coping strategies, *Family Relations*, 42(4): 383–91.

Kramer, B. and Vitaliano, P. (1994) Coping: a review of the theoretical frameworks and the measures used among caregivers of individuals with dementia, *Journal of Gerontological Social Work*, 23(1/2): 151–74.

Kresevic, D.M., Counsell, S.T., Covinsky, K. *et al.* (1998) A patient-centered model of acute care for elders, *Nursing Clinics of North America*, 33(3): 515–27.

Kropf, N.P. and Greene, R.R. (1993) Life review with families who care for developmentally disabled members: a model, *Journal of Gerontological Social Work*, 21(1/2): 25–40.

Krothe, J.S. (1997) Giving voice to elderly people: community-based long-term care, *Public Health Nursing*, 14(4): 217–26.

Kuhlman, G.J., Wilson, H.S., Hutchinson, S.A. and Wallhagen, M. (1991) Alzheimer's disease and family caregiving: critical synthesis of the literature and research agenda, *Nursing Research*, 40(6): 331–7.

Lafferty, G. (1996) Community based alternatives to hospital rehabilitation services: a review of the evidence and suggestions for approaching future evolution, *Reviews in Clinical Gerontology*, 6(2): 183–94.

Laing, W. (1998) *A Fair Price for Care? Disparities between Market Rates and State Funding of Residential Care.* York: York Publishing Services.

Laird, C. (1982) *Limbo: a Memoir of Life in a Nursing Home by a Survivor.* Novato, CA: Chandler and Sharp.

Lakhani, A. (1995) The role of outcomes assessment in improving clinical effectiveness, in M. Deighan and S. Hitch (eds) *Clinical Effectiveness from Guidelines to Cost-Effective Practice.* London: Department of Health.

Laman, H. and Lankhorst, G.J. (1994) Subjective weighting of disability: an approach to quality of life assessment in rehabilitation, *Disability and Rehabilitation*, 16(4): 198–204.

Lamb, G.S. and Stempel, J.E. (1994) Nurse case management from the client's view: growing as insider-expert, *Nursing Outlook*, 42: 7–13.

Landrum, P.K., Schmidt, N.D. and McLean, A.J. (1995) *Outcome Orientated Rehabilitation: Principles, Strategies and Tools for Effective Program Management.* Gaithersburg, MD: Aspen.

Laslett, P. (1989) *A Fresh Map of Life*. London: Weidenfeld and Nicolson.

Lauder, W. (1993) Health promotion in the elderly, *British Journal of Nursing*, 2(8): 401–4.

Lawlor, B. and Radic, A. (1994) Prevalence of mental illness in an elderly community dwelling population using Agecat, *Irish Journal of Psychological Medicine*, 11(4): 157–9.

Lawrence, J.A., Wearing, A.S. and Dodds, A.E. (1996) Nurses' representations of the positive and negative feature of nursing, *Journal of Advanced Nursing*, 24(2): 375–84.

Lawton, M.P. (1997) Quality of life. Keynote Presentation at Sixteenth Congress of the International Association of Gerontology, Adelaide.

Lawton, M.P., Moss, M. and Dunamel, L.M. (1995) The quality of life among elderly care receivers, *Journal of Applied Gerontology*, 14(2): 150–71.

Lea, A. (1994) Defining the roles of lay and nurse caring, *Nursing Standard*, 9(5): 32–5.

Lee-Treweek, G. (1994) Bedroom abuse: the hidden work in a nursing home, *Generations Review*, 4(2): 2–4.

Levine, M.E. (1995) The rhetoric of nursing theory, *Image: Journal of Nursing Scholarship*, 27(1): 11–14.

Levkoff, S.E., Macarthur, I.W. and Bucknall, J. (1995) Elderly mental health in the developing world, *Social Science and Medicine*, 41(7): 983–1003.

Lewis, J. and Meredith, B. (1988a) *Daughters Who Care: Daughters Caring for Mothers at Home*. London: Routledge and Kegan Paul.

Lewis, J. and Meredith, B. (1988b) Daughters caring for mothers, *Ageing and Society*, 8(1): 1–21.

Ley, D.C.H. (1989) The elderly and palliative care, *Journal of Palliative Care*, 5(4): 43–5.

Liaschenko, J. (1997) Knowing the patient, in S.E. Thorne and V.E. Hays (eds) *Nursing Praxis: Knowledge and Action*. Thousand Oaks, CA: Sage.

Liddle, J., Gilleard, C. and Neil, A. (1993) Elderly patients' and their relatives' views on CPR (letter). *Lancet*, 23 October: 1055.

Lifshitz, H. (1998) Instrumental enrichment: a tool for enrichment of cognitive ability in adult and elderly people with mental retardation, *Education and Training in Mental Retardation and Developmental Disabilities*, 33(1): 34–41.

Lindesay, J. (1991) Affective disorders in old age, *International Journal in Geriatric Psychiatry*, 124: 460–9.

Lindgren, C.L. (1993) The caregiver career. *Image: Journal of Nursing Scholarship*, 25(3): 214–19.

Liukkonen, A. (1995) Life in a nursing home for the frail elderly, *Clinical Nursing Research*, 4(4): 358–72.

Livingston, G., Watkin, V., Milne, B., Manela, M.V. and Katona, C. (1997) The natural history of depression and the anxiety disorders in older people: the Islington community study, *Journal of Affective Disorders*, 46: 255–62.

Livingston, G., Watkin, V. and Manela, M. (1998) Quality of life in older people, *Aging and Mental Health*, 2(1): 20–3.

Livneh, H. (1995) The tripartite model of rehabilitation interventions: basics, goals and rehabilitation strategies, *Journal of Applied Rehabilitation Counselling*, 26(1): 25–9.

Loew, F. and Rapin, C. (1994) The paradoxes of quality of life and its phenomenological approach, *Journal of Palliative Care*, 10(1): 37–41.

Lubinski, R. (1995) State-of-the-art perspectives on communication in nursing-homes, *Topics in Language Disorders*, 15(2): 1–19.

Luborsky, M.R. (1995) The process of self report of impairment in clinical research, *Social Science and Medicine*, 40(11): 1447–59.

Lundh, U. and Nolan, M.R. (1996) Ageing and quality of life 1: towards a better understanding, *British Journal of Nursing*, 5(20): 1248–51.

Lynn, J., Teno, J.M., Phillips, R.S. *et al.* (1997) Perceptions by family members of the dying experience of older and seriously ill patients. SUPPORT Investigators. Study to Understand Prognoses and Preferences for Outcomes and Risks of Treatments. *Annals of Internal Medicine*, 126(2): 97–106.

McCarthy, M., Addington-Hall, J.M. and Altmann, D. (1997) The experience of dying with dementia: a retrospective study, *International Journal of Geriatric Psychiatry*, 12: 404–9.

McColl, M.A. (1995) Social support, disability, and rehabilitation, *Critical Reviews in Physical and Rehabilitation Medicine*, 7(4): 315–33.

McCormack, B. and Ford, P. (1999a) Assessing older people's needs – a global challenge, *Ageing Matters*, spring/summer: 2–3.

McCormack, B. and Ford, P. (1999b) The contribution of expert gerontological nursing, *Nursing Standard*, 13(25): 42–5.

McCormack, B. and Wright, J. (1999) Achieving dignified care for older people through practice development: a systematic approach, *NT Research*, 4(5): 340–52.

McFadyn, J. and Farrington, A. (1997) User and carer participation in the NHS, *British Journal of Health Care Management*, 3(5): 260–4.

McFall, R.M. (1993) The essential role of theory in psychological assessment, in R.L. Gluekauf, L.B. Sechrest, G.R. Bond and E.G. McDaniel (eds) *Improving Assessment in Rehabilitation and Health*. Newbury Park, CA: Sage.

McGrath, M. and Grant, G. (1993) The life cycle and support networks of families with a person with a learning difficulty, *Disability, Handicap and Society*, 8(1): 25–41.

McGrother, C.W., Hauck, A., Bhaumik, S., Thorp, C. and Taub, N. (1996) Community care for adults with learning disability and their carers: needs and outcomes from the Leicester register, *Journal of Intellectual Disability Research*, 40: 183–90.

McGuire, B.E., Choon, G. and Akuffo, E. (1991) Community living for elderly people with an intellectual disability: a pilot study, *Australia and New Zealand Journal of Developmental Disabilities*, 17(1): 25–33.

Machell, S., Makenzie, K. and Phillips, W. (1988) Age well in Riverside, *Health Visitor*, 61: 21–2.

McNamara, B. (1997) A good enough death? Paper presented at the Social Context of Death, Dying and Disposal, Third International Conference, Cardiff University, April.

Maestri-Banks, A. and Gosney, M. (1997) Nurses' response to terminal care in the geriatric unit, *International Journal of Palliative Nursing*, 3(6): 345–50.

Mahoney, D.F. (1992) Hearing loss among nursing home residents: perceptions and realities, *Clinical Nursing Research*, 1(4): 317–32.

Malassiotis, A. and Newell, R. (1996) Nurses awareness of restraint use with elderly people in Greece and the UK: a cross-cultural study, *International Journal of Nursing Studies*, 33(2): 201–11.

Malin, N., Manthorpe, J. and Rose, D. (1999) *Community Care for Nurses and the Caring Professions*. Buckingham: Open University Press.

Marie Curie Memorial Foundation (1952) *Report of a National Survey concerning Patients with Cancer Nursed at Home*. London: Marie Curie Memorial Foundation.

Marr, J. (1994) The impact of HIV on older people: part 2, *Nursing Standard*, 8(47): 25–7.

Marris, V. (1996) *Lives Worth Living: Women's Experience of Chronic Illness*. London: Pandora.

Marshall, T. (1997) Infected and affected: HIV, AIDS and the older adult, *Generations Review*, 7(4): 9–11.

Martlew, B. (1996) What do you let the patient tell you?, *Physiotherapy*, 82(10): 558–65.

Mathers, C.D. and Robine, J.M. (1998) International trends in health expectations: a review. Thematic keynote highlights, 1997 World Congress of Gerontology, Ageing Beyond 2000. One World One Future, *Australian Journal on Ageing*, 17(1): 51–5.

Matsuda, O. (1994) Subjective burden of caregivers of demented patients – effects of coping and family adaptability, *Japanese Journal of Psychiatry and Neurology*, 48(4): 773–7.

Matthew, L. (1996) *Professional Care for the Elderly Mentally Ill*. London: Chapman and Hall.

Mattiasson, A.C. and Andersson, L. (1994) Staff attitude and experience in dealing with rational nursing home patients who refuse to eat and drink, *Journal of Advanced Nursing*, 20(5): 822–7.

Mayers, C.A. (1995) Defining and assessing quality of life. *British Journal of Occupational Therapy*, 58(4): 146–50.

Mechanic, D. (1995) Emerging trends in the application and social sciences to health and medicine, *Social Science and Medicine*, 11: 1491–6.

Mental Health Foundation (1995) *Making Life Better: Mental Health for Older People*. London: Mental Health Foundation.

Mezey, M.D., Lynaugh J.E. and Cartier, M.M. (1988) The Teaching Nursing Home Program, 1982–87: a report card, *Nursing Outlook*, 36(6): 285–9.

Miller, E.J. and Gwynne, G.V. (1972) *A Life Apart: a Pilot Study of Residential Institutions for the Physically Handicapped and the Young Chronic Sick*. London: Tavistock.

Milz, M. (1992) Healthy ill people: social cynicism or new perspectives, in A. Kaplun (ed.) *Health Promotion and Chronic Illness: Discovering a New Quality of Health*. Copenhagen: WHO Regional Publications.

Ministry of Health (1945) *Hospital Survey: the Hospital Services of Berkshire, Buckinghamshire and Oxfordshire*. London: HMSO.

Minkler, M. (1996) Critical perspectives on ageing: new challenges for gerontology, *Ageing and Society*, 16(4): 467–87.

Minkler, M. and Checkoway, B. (1998) Ten principles for geriatric health promotion, *Geriatric Health Promotion*, 3: 277–85.

Mitchell, P. and Koch, T. (1997) An attempt to give nursing home residents a voice in the quality improvement process: the challenge of frailty, *Journal of Clinical Nursing*, 6(6): 453–61.

Mogielnicki, R.P., Nelson, W.A. and Dulac, J. (1990) A study of the dying process in elderly hospitalised males, *Journal of Cancer Education*, 5(2): 135–45.

Mooney, R.P., Mooney, D.R. and Cohernour, K.L. (1995) Applied humanism: a model for managing inappropriate behaviour among mentally retarded elders, *Journal of Gerontological Nursing*, 21(8): 45–50.

Moore, T., Matyas, Y. and Boudreau, A. (1996) Describing and analyzing constipation in acute care, *Journal of Nursing Care Quality*, 10(3): 68–74.

Moos, R.H. and Schaefer, J.A. (eds) (1986) Coping with life crises: an integrated approach. New York: Plenum.

Morrell, J., Mernick, M., Brown, R. and Brooker, C. (1995) *Training Needs Assessment of Qualified Nurses in Private Nursing Homes in Trent*. Sheffield: School of Health and Related Research, University of Sheffield.

Morris, J. and Bowman, C. (1999) Community institutional healthcare: emergence from refugee status, *Journal of the Royal Society of Medicine*, 92(6): 271–2.

Morriss, R.K., Rovner, B.W. and German, P.S. (1995) Clinical and psychosocial variables associated with different types of behavior problem in new nursing-home admissions, *International Journal of Geriatric Psychiatry*, 10(7): 547–55.

Morrow, E. (1997) Attitudes of women from vulnerable populations to physician and assisted death, *Journal of Clinical Ethics*, 8(3): 279–89.

Morrow-Howell, N. (1998) Building bridges between families and nursing home staff: the Partners in Caregiving program, *Gerontologist*, 38(4): 499–503.

Morse, J., Bottorff, J. and Hutchinson, S. (1994) The phenomenology of comfort, *Journal of Advanced Nursing*, 20: 189–95.

Moss, S. (1991) Age and functional abilities of people with a mental handicap: evidence from the Wessex mental handicap register, *Journal of Mental Deficiency Research*, 35: 430–45.

Moss, S. and Patel, P. (1993) The prevalence of mental illness in people with intellectual disability over 50 years of age and the diagnostic importance of information from carers, *Irish Journal of Psychology*, 14: 110–29.

Motenko, A.K. (1989) The frustrations, gratifications and well-being of dementia caregivers, *Gerontologist*, 29(2): 166–72.

Mount, B. (1989) cited in D.P. Ryan, M.G. Carson and M.L. Zorzitto (1989) The first international conference on the palliative care of the elderly: an overview, *Journal of Palliative Care*, 5(4): 40–2.

Mulkay, M. (1993) Social death in Britain, in D. Clark (ed.) *The Sociology of Death*. Oxford: Basil Blackwell.

Mulrooney, C.P. (1997) Competencies needed by formal caregivers to enhance elders' quality of life: the unitility of the 'Person – and Relationship-Centred Caregiving (PRCC) Trait'. Sixteenth Congress of the International Association of Gerontology, Adelaide.

Murphy, E. (1988) Prevention of depression and suicide, in B. Gearing, M. Johnson and T. Heller (eds) *Mental Health Problems in Old Age*. Chichester: Wiley.

Murphy, J.F. and Hepworth, J.T. (1996) Age and gender differences in health services utilization, *Research in Nursing and Health*, 19: 323–9.

Murphy, K., Hanrahan, P. and Luchins, D. (1997) A survey of grief and bereavement in nursing homes: the importance of hospice grief and bereavement for the end-stage Alzheimer's disease patient and family, *Journal of the American Geriatrics Society*, 45(9): 1104–7.

Naleppa, M.J. (1996) Families and the institutionalised elderly: a review, *Journal of Gerontological Social Work*, 27(1/2): 87–111.

National Council for Hospice and Specialist Palliative Care Services (NCHSPCS) (1993) *Key Ethical Issues in Palliative Care. Evidence to the House of Lords Select Committee on Medical Ethics, occasional paper no. 3*. London: NCHSPCS.

National Council for Hospice and Specialist Palliative Care Services (NCHSPCS) (1997) *Voluntary Euthanasia: the Council's View*. London: NCHSPCS.

Nay, R. (1995) Nursing home residents' perceptions of relocation, *Journal of Clinical Nursing*, 4(5): 319–25.

Nay, R. (1999) Issues in gerontic nursing in Australia, in S.H. Gueldner and L.W. Poon (eds) *Gerontological Nursing Issues for the Twenty-First Century*. Indianapolis, IN: Sigma Theta Tau International.

Nay, R. and Closs, B. (1999) Staffing and quality in non-acute facilities, in R. Nay and S. Garret (eds) *Nursing Older People: Issues and Innovations*. Sydney: Maclennan and Petty.

Nazarko, L. (1998) Quality of care in nursing homes, *Nursing Management*, 5(8): 17–20.

Neil, R., Casey, T. and Kennedy, M. (1982) Nursing homes for initial clinical experience: some specific advantages, *Nursing and Health Care*, 3: 319–23.

NHS Confederation and the Sainsbury Centre for Mental Health (1997) *The Way Forward for Mental Health Services*. London: HMSO.

NHS Executive (1998) *Signposts for Success in Commissioning and Providing Health Services for People with Learning Disabilities*. Wetherby: NHS Executive.

Nilsson, M., Ekman, S-L., Ericsson, K. and Winblad, B. (1996) Some characteristics of the quality of life in old age illustrated by means of Allardt's Concept, *Scandinavian Journal of Caring Sciences*, 10(2): 116–21.

Nilsson, M., Ekman, S. and Sarvimäki, A. (1998) Ageing with joy or resigning to old age: older people's experiences of the quality of life in old age, *Health Care in Later Life*, 3(2): 94–110.

Nkongo, N.O. and Archbold, P.G. (1995) Reasons for caregiving in African American families, *Journal of Cultural Diversity*, 2(4): 116–23.

Nocon, A. and Baldwin, S. (1998) *Towards a Rehabilitation Policy: a Review of the Literature*. London: King's Fund.

Nocon, A. and Qureshi, U. (1996) *Outcomes of Community Care for Users and Carers: A Social Services Perspective*. Buckingham: Open University Press.

Nolan, M.R. (1997) Health and social care: what the future holds for nursing. Keynote address at Third Royal College of Nursing Older Person European Conference and Exhibition, Harrogate.

Nolan, M.R. and Caldock, K. (1996) Assessment: identifying the barriers to good practice, *Health and Social Care in the Community*, 4(2): 77–85.

Nolan, M. and Dellasega, C. (1999) 'It's not the same as him being at home': creating caring partnerships following nursing home placement, *Journal of Clinical Nursing*, 8: 723–30.

Nolan, M.R. and Grant, G. (1992a) Helping new carers of the frail elderly patient: the challenge for nursing in acute care settings, *Journal of Clinical Nursing*, 1: 303–7.

Nolan, M.R. and Grant, G. (1992b) *Regular Respite: an Evaluation of a Hospital Rota Bed Scheme for Elderly People*. London: Age Concern.

Nolan, M. and Grant, G. (1993) Rust out and therapeutic reciprocity: concepts to advance the nursing care of older people, *Journal of Advanced Nursing*, 18: 1305–14.

Nolan, M.R. and Keady, J. (1996) Training in long-term care: the road to better quality, *Reviews in Clinical Gerontology*, 6: 333–42.

Nolan, M., Grant, G. and Nolan, J. (1995a) Busy doing nothing: activity and interaction levels amongst differing populations of elderly patients, *Journal of Advanced Nursing*, 22(3): 528–38.

Nolan, M.R., Grant, G. and Keady, J. (1996a) *Understanding Family Care*. Buckingham: Open University Press.

Nolan, M., Keady, J. and Grant, G. (1995b) CAMI: a basis for assessment and support with family carers, *British Journal of Adult/Elderly Care Nursing*, 1(3): 822–6.

Nolan, M., Walker, G., Nolan, J. *et al.* (1996b) Entry to care: positive choice or fait accompli? Developing a more proactive nursing response to the needs of older people and their carers, *Journal of Advanced Nursing*, 24(2): 265–74.

Nolan, M.R., Nolan, J. and Booth, A. (1997) Preparation for multi-professional/multi-agency health care practice: the nursing contribution to rehabilitation within the multidisciplinary team, literature review and curriculum analysis. Final Report to the English National Board. Sheffield: University of Sheffield.

Nolan, M.R., Grant, G. and Keady, J. (1998b) *Assessing the Needs of Family Carers: a Guide for Practitioners*. Brighton: Pavilion.

Nolan, M., Lundh, L. and Tishelman, C. (1998c) Nursing knowledge: does it have to be unique? *British Journal of Nursing*, 7(5): 270–6.

Nolan, M.R., Grant, S., Brown, J. and Nolan, J. (1998a) Assessing nurses' work environment: old dilemmas, new solutions, *Clinical Effectiveness in Nursing*, 2: 145–56.

Nolan, P., Badger, F. and Dunn, L. (1999a) Brainstorming the role of mental health nursing, *Nursing Times*, 17(4): 52–4.

Nolan, P., Murray, E. and Dallender, J. (1999b) Practice nurses' perceptions of services for clients with psychological problems in primary care, *International Journal of Nursing Studies*, 36(2): 97–104.

Norburn, J.E.K., Nettles-Carlson, B., Soltys, F.G., Read, C.D. and Pickard, C.G. (1995) Long-term care organizational challenges and strategies: art vs. regulation, *Journal of Gerontological Nursing*, 21(8): 37–44, 54–5.

Norman, I.J. and Redfern, S.J. (1997) *Mental Health Care for Elderly People*. Edinburgh: Churchill Livingstone.

Nystrom, A. and Segesten, K. (1990) Peace of mind as an important aspect of old people's health, *Scandinavian Journal of Caring Sciences*, 4(2): 55–62.

Nystrom, A.E. and Segesten, K.M. (1994) On sources of powerlessness in nursing home life, *Journal of Advanced Nursing*, 19(1): 124–33.

Nystrom, A.E. and Segesten, K.M. (1995) Support of the experience of health in lucid elderly nursing home patients: registered nurses' perceptions, *Scandinavian Journal of Caring Sciences*, 9(3): 145–52.

O'Boyle, C.A. (1997) Measuring the quality of later life, *Philosophical Transactions of the Royal Society of London Series B-Biological Sciences*, 352(136): 1871–9.

O'Brien, J. (1994) Down stairs that are never your own: supporting people with developmental disabilities in their own homes, *Mental Retardation*, 32: 1–6.

O'Brien, J. and O'Brien, C.L. (1991) *Framework for Accomplishments*, Georgia: Responsive Service Systems.

Ogg, J., Evans, J.G., Jelterys, M. and MacMahon, D.G. (1998) Professional responses to the challenge of old age, in M. Bernard and J. Phillips (eds) *The Social Policy of Old Age: Moving into the 21st Century*. London: Centre for Policy on Ageing.

Oleson, M. and Shadick, K.M. (1993) Application of Moos and Schaefer's (1986) model to nursing care of elderly persons relocating to a nursing home, *Journal of Advanced Nursing*, 18(3): 479–85.

Oleson, M., Heading, C., McGlynn Shadick, K. and Bistodeau, J.A. (1994) Quality of life in long-stay institutions in England: nurse and resident perceptions, *Journal of Advanced Nursing*, 20: 23–32.

Oliver, M. (1993) A different view: who needs rehabilitating, in R. Greenwood, M.P. Barnes, T.M. McMillan and C.O. Vord (eds) *Neurological Rehabilitation*. Edinburgh: Churchill Livingstone.

Oliver, M. (1996) *Understanding Disability*. London: Macmillan.

Olsson, E. and Ingvad, B. (1999) The emotional climate of the caring relationship in home care services. Paper presented at the Fourth European Congress of Gerontology, 7–11 July, Berlin.

Ory, M.G. and Williams, F. (1989) Rehabilitation: small goals, sustained interventions, *Annals of the American Academy of Political and Social Science*, 503: 60–71.

Osberg, J., Mcginnis, G.E., DeJong, G. and Seward, M.L. (1987) Life satisfaction and quality of life among disabled elderly adults, *Journal of Gerontology*, 42: 228–30.

Pabst-Battin, M. (1994) *The Least Worst Death: Essays in Bioethics on the End of Life*. Oxford: Oxford University Press.

Pahl, R. (1999) Social trends: the social context of healthy living, *Policy futures for UK health no. 6*. London: Nuffield Trust.

Palat, M. (1992) The triangulation model of rehabilitation medicine, *European Rehabilitation*, 2: 85–7.

Paley, J. (1996) Intuition and expertise: comments on the Benner debate, *Journal of Advanced Nursing*, 22: 40–7.

Parkes, L. (1992) Pain amongst cognitively impaired elderly, *Canadian Nurse*, 88(7): 20–2.

Parrott, R., Emerson, E., Hatton, C. and Wolstenholme, J. (1997) *Future Demand for Residential Provision for People with Learning Disabilities*. Manchester: Hester Adrian Research Centre.

Patchner, M.A. and Patchner, L.S. (1993) Essential staffing for improved nursing home care: the permanent assignment model, *Nursing Homes*, 42(5): 37–9.

Patel, P., Goldberg, D. and Moss, S. (1993) Psychiatric morbidity in older people with moderate and severe learning disabilities: the prevalence study, *British Journal of Psychiatry*, 163: 481–91.

Patterson, B.J. (1995) The process of social support: adjusting to life in a nursing home, *Journal of Advanced Nursing*, 21(4): 682–9.

Pawlson, L.G. (1994) Health care reform: chronic illness – implications of a new paradigm for health care, *Joint Commission Journal on Quality Improvement*, 20(1): 33–9.

Pearson, A., Hocking, S., Mott, S. and Rigg, A. (1992) Skill mix in Australian nursing homes, *Journal of Advanced Nursing*, 17: 767–76.

Pearson, A., Nay, R., Taylor, B. *et al.* (1998) *Relatives' Experiences of Nursing Home Entry: Meanings, Practices and Discourses. Second Interim Report, Research Monograph Series no. 4*. Adelaide: University of Adelaide.

Peate, I. (1999) The need to address sexuality in older people, *British Journal of Community Nursing*, 4(4): 174–9.

Peressini, T. and McDonald, L. (1998) An evaluation of a training program on alcoholism and older adults for health care and social service, *Gerontology and Geriatrics Education*, 18(4): 23–44.

Perry, L. (1997) Nutrition: a hard nut to crack. An exploration of the knowledge, attitudes and activities of qualified nurses in relation to nutritional nursing care, *Journal of Clinical Nursing*, 6(4): 315–24.

Peters, D.J. (1995) Human experience in disablement: the impetus of the ICIDH, *Disability and Rehabilitation*, 17(3214): 135–44.

Phillipson, C. and Biggs, S. (1998) Modernity and identity: theories and perspectives in the study of older adults, *Journal of Aging and Identity*, 3(1): 11–23.

Phillipson, C.A. and Strang, P. (1985) Training for health education with older people: a survey of district nurse and health visitor courses, *Nurse Education Today*, 5(6): 247–51.

Philp, I. (1996) Comment community alternatives to hospital care, *Reviews in Clinical Gerontology*, 6: 195–6.

Philp, I., Ashe, A. and Lothian, K. (2000) Designing and implementing service frameworks in the NHS, in A. Warnes, L. Warren and M. Nolan (eds) *Care Services for Later Life: Transformations and Critiques*. London: Jessica Kingsley.

Pincombe, J., O'Brien, B., Cleek, J. and Ballantyre, A. (1996) Critical aspects of nursing in aged and extended care, *Journal of Advanced Nursing*, 23(4): 672–8.

Poon, L.W. and Gueldner, S.H. (1999) An essay reflection on the International Year of Older Persons, in S.H. Guelner and L.W. Poon (eds) *Gerontological Nursing Issues for the Twenty-First Century*. Indianapolis, IN: Sigma Theta Tau International.

Porter, E. (1995) A phenomenological alternative to the 'ADL Research Tradition', *Journal of Aging and Health*, 7(1): 24–45.

Pot, A. and Deeg, D. (1998) Psychological distress of caregivers: the mediator effect of caregiving appraisal, *Patient Education and Counselling*, 34(1): SISI, 43–51.

Powell, C. and Crombie, A. (1974) The Kilsyth Questionnaire: a method of screening elderly people at home, *Age and Ageing*, 3: 23–8.

Powell-Lawton, M. (1997) Measures of quality of life and subjective well-being, *Generations*, XXI(1): 45–7.

Powers, B.A. (1991) The meaning of nursing home friendships, *Advances in Nursing Science*, 14(2): 42–58.

Powers, B.A. (1992) The roles staff play in the social networks of elderly institutionalized people, *Social Science and Medicine*, 34(12): 1335–43.

Poxton, R. (1998) Community care for older people: taking the broad view for radical change, *Managing Community Care*, 6(1): 13–19.

Prager, E. (1997) Sources of personal meaning in life for a sample of younger and older urban Australian women, *Journal of Women and Aging*, 9(3): 47–65.

Prasher, V. (1995) Age specific prevalence, thyroid dysfunction and depressive symptomatology in adults with Down syndrome and dementia, *International Journal of Geriatric Psychiatry*, 10: 25–31.

Prince, M. (1985) The challenge of our age, *Periodical on Ageing*, 1(1): 2–15.

Proctor, R., Stratton Powell, H., Burns, A. *et al.* (1998) An observational study to evaluate the impact of a specialist outreach team on the quality of care in nursing and residential homes, *Aging and Mental Health*, 2(3): 232–8.

Prophet, H. (ed.) (1998) *Fit for the Future: the Prevention of Dependency in Later Life*. London: Continuing Care Conference.

Prosser, H. (1997) The future care plans of older adults with intellectual disabilities living at home with family carers, *Journal of Applied Research in Intellectual Disabilities*, 10(1): 15–32.

Prosser, H. and Moss, S. (1996) Informal care networks of older adults with an intellectual disability, *Journal of Applied Research in Intellectual Disabilities*, 9(1): 17–30.

Pursey, A. and Luker, K. (1993) Assessment of older people at home, in J. Wilson-Barnett and J. Macleod-Clark (eds) *Research in Health Promotion and Nursing*. London: Macmillan.

Quinn, A.A., Barton, J.A. and Magilvy, J.K. (1995) Weathering the storm: metaphors and stories of living with multiple sclerosis, *Rehabilitation Nursing Research*, 4: 19–27.

Racino, J.A. and Heumann, J.E. (1992) Independent living and community life:

building coalitions among elders, people with disabilities, and our allies, *Generations*, winter: 43–7.

Ragneskog, H., Kihlgren, M., Karlsson, I. and Norberg, A. (1996) Dinner music for demented patients: analysis of video-recorded observations, *Clinical Nursing Research*, 5(3): 262–82.

Ragneskog, H., Gerdner, L.A., Josefsson, K. and Kihlgren, M. (1998) Probable reasons for expressed agitation in persons with dementia, *Clinical Nursing Research*, 7(2): 189–206.

Raynes, N.V. (1998) Involving residents in quality specification, *Ageing and Society*, 18(1): 65–77.

Redfern, S. (1999) Older people and therapeutic care, *Journal of Clinical Nursing*, 8: 327–8.

Redfern, S. and Norman, I. (1999) Quality of nursing care perceived by patients and their nurses: an application of the clinical incident technique: parts 1 and 2, *Journal of Clinical Nursing*, 8: 407–21.

Reece, A.C. and Simpson, J.M. (1996) Preparing older people to cope after a fall, *Physiotherapy*, 82(4): 227–35.

Reed, J. (1998) Gerontological nursing research – future directions. Paper given to the Agenet/Royal College of Nursing gerontological nursing research seminar, Regents College, London, December.

Reed, J. and Bond, S. (1991) Nurses' assessment of elderly patients in hospital, *International Journal of Nursing Studies*, 28(1): 55–64.

Reed, J. and Clarke, C.L. (1999a) Nursing older people: considering need and care, *Nursing Inquiry*, 6: 208–15.

Reed, J. and Clarke, C. (1999b) Older people with mental health problems: maintaining a dialogue, in M. Clinton and S. Nelson (eds) *Advanced Practice in Mental Health Nursing*. Oxford: Blackwell Science.

Reed, J. and Payton, V.R. (1998) Understanding the dynamics of life in care homes for older people: implications for de-institutionalising practice, *Health and Social Care in the Community*, 5(4): 261–8.

Reed, J. and Watson, D. (1994) The impact of the medical model on nursing practice and assessment, *International Journal of Nursing Studies*, 21(1): 57–66.

Reed, J., Roskell Payton, V. and Bond, S. (1998) The importance of place for older people moving into care homes, *Social Science and Medicine*, 46(7): 859–67.

Reed, J., Cook, G. and Stanley, D. (1999) Promoting partnership with older people through quality assurance systems: issues arising in care homes, *NT Research*, 4(5): 353–63.

Relatives' Association (1997) *As Others See Us: a Study of Relationships in Homes for Older People*. London: Relatives' Association.

Renwick, R. and Brown, I. (1996) The Centre for Health Practitioners: conceptual approach to quality of life – being, belonging and becoming, in R. Renwick, I. Brown and M. Nagler (eds) *Quality of Life in Health Promotion: Conceptual Approaches, Issues and Applications*. Thousand Oaks, CA: Sage.

Renwick, R. and Friefild, S. (1996) Quality of life and rehabilitation, in R. Renwick, I. Brown and M. Nagler (eds) *Quality of Life in Health Promotion and Rehabilitation: Conceptual Approaches, Issues and Applications*. Thousand Oaks, CA: Sage.

Renwick, R., Brown, I. and Nagler, M. (eds) (1996) *Quality of Life in Health Promotion and Rehabilitation: Conceptual Approaches, Issues and Applications*. Thousand Oaks, CA: Sage.

Repper, J., Brooker, C. and Repper, D. (1995) Serious mental health problems: policy changes, *Nursing Times*, 91(25): 29–31.

Resnick, B., Slocum, D., Ra, L. and Moffett, P. (1996) Geriatric rehabilitation: nursing interventions and outcomes focusing on urinary function and knowledge of medications, *Rehabilitation Nursing*, 21(3): 142–7.

Reynolds, C. (1992) An administrative program to facilitate culturally appropriate care for the elderly, *Holistic Nursing Practice*, 6(3): 34–42.

Rhodes, P. and Shaw, S. (1999) Informal care and terminal illness, *Health and Social Care in the Community*, 7(1): 39–50.

Richmond, D. and McCracken, H. (1996) Health promotion and education for the elderly: experience in an academic department of geriatric medicine, *Australian Journal on Ageing*, 15(1): 18–21.

Rickard, W. (1995) HIV/AIDS and older people, *HIV/AIDS and Older People*, 5(3): 2–6.

Robb, B. (1967) *Sans Everything: a Case to Answer*. London: Nelson.

Roberto, K.A. (1993) Family caregivers of ageing adults with disabilities, in K.A. Roberto (ed.) *The Elderly Caregiver: Caring for Adults with Developmental Disabilities*. Newbury Park, CA: Sage.

Robertson, J., Moss, S. and Turner, S. (1996) Policy, services and staff training for older people with intellectual disability in the UK, *Journal of Applied Research in Intellectual Disabilities*, 9(2): 91–100.

Robinson, C. and Williams, V. (1999) *In their Own Right*. Bristol: Norah Fry Research Centre, Bristol University.

Robinson, I. (1988) The rehabilitation of patients with long term physical impairments: the social context of professional roles, *Clinical Rehabilitation*, 2: 339–47.

Robinson, J. and Batstone, G. (1996) *Rehabilitation: a Development Challenge*. London: King's Fund.

Rodwell, C.M. (1996) An analysis of the concept of empowerment, *Journal of Advanced Nursing*, 23(2): 305–13.

Rohde, J., Farmer, R. and McCarthy, J. (1995) Elderly people with learning disability: a comparison of people over the age of 61 in 1984 and those over the age of 61 in 1994, *British Journal of Learning Disabilities*, 23: 143–6.

Rolland, J.S. (1994) *Families, Illness and Disability: an Integrative Treatment Model*. New York: Basic Books.

Ross, M.M., Rosenthal, C.J. and Dawson, P. (1997) Spousal caregiving in the institutional setting: visiting, *Journal of Clinical Nursing*, 6(6): 473–83.

Roth, M. (1996) Euthanasia and related ethical issues in dementias of later life with special reference to Alzheimer's disease, *British Medical Bulletin*, 52(2): 263–79.

Rowntree, S. (1947) *Old People: Report of a Survey Committee on the Problems of Ageing and the Care of Old People Under the Chairmanship of Seebohm Rowntree*. London: The Nuffield Foundation.

Royal College of Nursing (1992) *A Scandal Waiting to Happen?* London: Royal College of Nursing.

Royal College of Nursing (1994) *An Inspector Calls: the Regulation of Private Nursing Homes and Hospitals*. London: Royal College of Nursing.

Royal Commission on Long-Term Care (1999) *With Respect to Old Age*. London: The Stationery Office.

Ruland, C.M., Kresevic, D. and Lorenson, M. (1997) Including patient preferences in nurses' assessment of older patients, *Journal of Clinical Nursing*, 6(6): 495–504.

Ruth, J.E. and Öberg, P. (1996) Ways of life: old age in a life history perspective, in

J.E. Birren, G.M. Kenyon, J.E. Ruth, J.J.F. Schroots and T. Svensomm (eds) *Ageing and Biography: Explorations in Adult Development*. New York: Springer.

Ryle, G. (1949) *The Concept of Mind*. London: Hutchinson.

Sachs, G.A., Ahronheim, J.C., Rhymes, J.A., Volicer, L. and Lynn, J. (1995) Good care of dying patients: the alternative to physician assisted suicide and euthanasia, *Journal of the American Geriatric Society*, 43(5): 553–62.

Salgado, R., Ehrlich, F., Banks, C. *et al*. (1995) A mobile rehabilitation team program to assist patients in nursing-homes rehabilitate and return to their homes, *Archives of Gerontology and Geriatrics*, 20(3): 255–61.

Sällström, C. (1994) Spouses' experiences of living with a partner with Alzheimer's disease. Unpublished PhD thesis, Department of Advanced Nursing, Geriatric Medicine and Psychiatry, University of Umeå, Sweden.

Salzman, C. (1997) Depressive disorders and other emotional issues in the elderly: current issues, *International Clinical Psychopharmacology*, 12(suppl. 7): 37–42.

Saunders, C. and Baines, M. (1983) *Living with Dying: the Management of Terminal Disease*. Oxford: Oxford University Press.

Saunders, C., Summers, D. and Teller, N. (1981) *Hospice: the Living Idea*. Leeds: Edward Arnold.

Saunders, P.A. (1989) Alcohol use and abuse in the elderly: findings from the Liverpool longitudinal study of continuing health in the community, *International Journal of Geriatric Psychiatry*, 4(2): 103–8.

Savishinsky, J.S. (1991) *The Ends of Time: Life and Work in a Nursing Home*. New York: Bergin and Garvey.

Scheidt, R.J., Humphreys, D.R. and Yorgason, J.B. (1999) Successful ageing: what's not to like?, *Journal of Applied Gerontology*, 18(8): 277–82.

Schön, D. (1987) *Educating the Reflective Practitioner*. San Francisco, CA: Jossey Bass.

Schonwetter, R.S. (1996) Care of the dying geriatric patient, *Clinics in Geriatric Medicine*, 10(2): 253–65.

Schultz, A., Dickey, G. and Skoner, M. (1997) Self-report of incontinence in acute care, *Journal of Urological Nursing*, 17(1): 23–8.

Schulz, R. and Williamson, G.M. (1993) Psychological and behavioural dimensions of physical frailty, *Journal of Gerontology*, 48(special edn): 39–43.

Schumacher, K.L., Stewart, B.J. and Archbold, P.G. (1998) Conceptualisation and measurement of doing family caregiving well, *Image: Journal of Nursing Scholarship*, 30(1): 63–70.

Seale, C. (1991) Death from cancer and death from other causes: the relevance of the hospice approach, *Palliative Medicine*, 5: 12–19.

Seale, C. (1996) Living alone towards the end of life, *Ageing and Society*, 16(1): 75–91.

Seale, C.F. and Addington-Hall, J.M. (1994) Euthanasia: why people want to die earlier, *Social Science and Medicine*, 39: 647–54.

Seale, C.F. and Addington-Hall, J.M. (1995) Dying at the best time, *Social Science and Medicine*, 40: 589–95.

Seale, C. and Cartwright, A. (1994) *The Year before Death*. Aldershot: Avebury.

Secker, J., Pidd, F. and Paraham, A. (1999) Mental health training needs of primary health care nurses, *Journal of Clinical Nursing*, 8(6): 643–52.

Select Committee on Medical Ethics (1994) *Report*. London: HMSO.

Seltzer, M.M. (1992) Training families to be case managers for elders with developmental disabilities, *Generations*, winter: 65–70.

Seltzer, M.M. and Krauss, M.W. (1989) Ageing parents with mentally retarded children: family risk factors and sources of support, *American Journal on Mental Retardation*, 94: 303–12.

Seltzer, M.M., Krauss, M.W. and Heller, T. (1991) Family caregiving over the life course, in M. Janicki and M.M. Seltzer (eds) *Proceedings of the Boston Roundtable on Research Issues and Applications in Ageing and Developmental Disabilities*. Boston, MA: American Associates on Mental Deficiency (AAMD).

Seymour, J.E. and Ingleton, C. (1999) Ethical issues in qualitative research at the end of life, *International Journal of Palliative Care Nursing*, 5(2): 65–73.

Sheldon, J.H. (1948) *The Social Medicine of Old Age: Report of an Inquiry in Wolverhampton*. London: Nuffield Foundation.

Siddell, M., Katz, J.T. and Komaromy, C. (1998) Death and dying in residential and nursing homes for older people. Unpublished report to the Department of Health.

Simon, J.M. (1996) Chronic pain syndrome: nursing assessment and intervention, *Rehabilitation Nursing*, 21(1): 13–19.

Sinclair, A. and Dickinson, E. (1998) *Effective Practice in Rehabilitation: the Evidence of Systematic Reviews*. London: King's Fund.

Sixsmith, A., Hawley, C., Stilwell, J. and Copeland, J. (1993) Delivering positive care in nursing-homes, *International Journal of Geriatric Psychiatry*, 8(5): 407–12.

Skilbeck, J., Mott, L., Smith, D., Page, H. and Clark, D. (1998) Nursing care for people dying from chronic obstructive airways disease, *International Journal of Palliative Nursing*, 3(2): 100–6.

Smith, A.M. (1994) Euthanasia present law protects doctors and patients (letter), *British Medical Journal*, 309: 471.

Smith, M., Buckwalter, K.C., Garand, L. *et al.* (1994) Evaluation of a geriatric mental health training program for nursing personnel in rural long-term care facilities, *Issues in Mental Health Nursing*, 15(2): 149–68.

Smith, M., Mitchell, S. and Buckwalter, K.C. (1995) Nurses helping nurses: development of internal specialists in long-term care, *Journal of Psychosocial Nursing and Mental Health Services*, 33(4): 38–42.

Smith, N. (1997) The role of continence promotion in rehabilitation, *Reviews in Clinical Gerontology*, 7(3): 257–64.

Smyer, M.A. and Qualls, S.H. (1999) *Aging and Mental Health*. London: Blackwell.

Snowdon, J. (1998) Management of late-life depression, *Australian Journal of Ageing*, 17(2): 57–62.

Snyder, L. (1999) *Speaking our Minds: Personal Reflections from Individuals with Alzheimer's Disease*. New York: Freeman.

Social Services Inspectorate (1995) *A Way Ahead for Carers: Priorities for Managers and Practitioners*. London: Social Services Inspectorate.

Social Services Inspectorate (1997) *The Cornerstone of Care: Inspection of Care Planning for Older People*. London: Department of Health.

Spaid, W.M. and Barusch, A.S. (1994) Emotional closeness and caregiver burden in marital relationship, *Journal of Gerontological Social Work*, 21(3/4): 197–211.

Spencer, J., Young, M.E., Rintala, D. and Bates, S. (1995) Socialisation to the culture of a rehabilitation hospital: an ethnographic study, *American Journal of Occupational Therapy*, 29(1): 35–62.

Spencer, J., Davidson, H. and White, V. (1997) Helping clients develop hopes for the future, *American Journal of Occupational Therapy*, 51(3): 191–8.

Standing Medical Advisory Committee (SMAC) and Standing Nursing and Midwifery Advisory Committee (SNMAC) (1992) *The Principles and Provision of Palliative Care*. London: HMSO.

Stedman, T. (1996) Approaches to measuring quality of life and their relevance to mental health, *Australian and New Zealand Journal of Psychiatry*, 30(6): 731–40.

Stevens, A.B., Burgio, L.D., Bailey, E. *et al.* (1998) Teaching and maintaining behaviour management skills with assistants in a nursing home. *Gerontologist*, 38(3): 379–84.

Stevens, J. (1997) The education and socialisation of nurses: why a carer with the elderly is a most unpopular career destination. Paper given at the Sixteenth World Congress of Gerontology, Adelaide.

Stevens, J. (1999) Ageism and economic fundamentalism, in R. Nay and G. Garrat (eds) *Nursing Older People, Issues and Innovations*. Sydney: Maclennan and Petty.

Stevenson, J.P. (1990) Family stress related to home care of Alzheimer's disease patients and implications for support, *Journal of Neuroscience Nursing*, 22(3): 179–88.

Steverink, N., Lindeiberg, S. and Ornel, J. (1998) Towards understanding successful ageing: patterned changes in resources and goals, *Ageing and Society*, 18(4): 441–68.

Stewart, B.J., Archbold, P.G., Harvath, T.A. and Nkongho, N.O. (1993) Role acquisition in family caregivers of older people who have been discharged from hospital, in S.G. Funk, E.H. Tornquist, M.T. Champagne and R.A. Weise (eds) *Key Aspects of Caring for the Chronically Ill: Hospital and Home*. New York: Springer.

Stoats, A., Heaphey, K., Miller, D. *et al.* (1993) Subjective age and health perceptions of older persons: maintaining the youthful bias in sickness and in health, *International Journal of Aging and Human Development*, 37(3): 191–203.

Stokes, S. (1994) *Health Visitors' Perceptions of their Role in Prevention of Accidents in the Elderly*. London: King's College, University of London.

Stover, S.L. (1995) Review of forty years of rehabilitation issues in spinal cord injury, *Journal of Spinal Cord Medicine*, 18: 175–82.

Strauss, A.L. and Corbin, J.M. (1988) *Shaping a New Health Care System: the Experience of Chronic Illness as a Catalyst for Change*. San Francisco, CA: Jossey Bass.

Strauss, A.L., Corbin, J.M., Fagerhaugh, S. *et al.* (1984) *Chronic Illness and the Quality of Life*. St Louis, MO: Mosby.

Studenski, S. and Duncan, P.W. (1993) Measuring rehabilitation outcomes: geriatric rehabilitation, *Clinics in Geriatric Medicine*, 9(11): 823–30.

Stumer, J., Hickson, L. and Worrall, L. (1996) Hearing impairment, disability and handicap in elderly people living in residential care and in the community, *Disability and Rehabilitation*, 18(2): 76–82.

Sudnow, D. (1967) *Passing On: the Social Organization of Dying*. Englewood Cliffs, NJ: Prentice Hall.

Swain, J. and French, J. (1998) Normality and disabling care, in A. Brechin, J. Walmsley, J. Katz and S. Peace (eds) *Care Matters: Concepts, Practice and Research in Health and Social Care*. London: Sage.

Sweeting, H. and Gilhoolhy, M. (1997) Dementia and the phenomenon of social death, *Sociology of Health and Illness*, 19(1): 93–117.

Swift, C.G. (1996) Disease and disability in older people: prospects for intervention, in A.J. Squires (ed.) *Rehabilitation of Older People: a Handbook for the MDT*. London: Chapman and Hall.

Taival, A. and Raatikainen, R. (1993) Finnish nursing homes: client well-being and staff development, *Journal of Gerontological Nursing*, 19(2): 19–24.

Takashida, S., Iida, K., Mito, T. and Arima, M. (1994) Dendritic and histochemical development and ageing in patients with Down's syndrome, *Journal of Intellectual Disability Research*, 38: 265–73.

Tallis, R. (1989) Measurement and the future of rehabilitation, *Geriatric Medicine*, 19(1): 31–40.

Tallis, R. (1992) Rehabilitation of the elderly in the 21st century, *Journal of Royal College of Physicians*, 26(4): 413–22.

Tang, S.Y.S. and Anderson, J.M. (1999) Human agency and the process of healing: lessons learned from women living with chronic illness: 're-writing the concept of expert', *Nursing Inquiry*, 6: 83–93.

Tanner, C.A., Benner, P., Chesla, C. and Gordon, D. (1996) The phenomenology of knowing the patient, in S. Gordon, P. Benner and N. Noddings (eds) *Caregiving: Readings in Knowledge, Practice, Ethics and Politics*. Philadelphia, PA: University of Pennsylvania Press.

Taraborrelli, P. (1993) Exemplar A: becoming a carer, in N. Gilbert (ed.) *Researching Social Life*. London: Sage.

Tarlow, B. (1996) Caring: a negotiated process that varies, in S. Gordon, P. Benner and N. Noddings (eds) *Caregiving: Readings in Knowledge, Practice, Ethics and Politics*. Philadelphia, PA: University of Pennsylvania Press.

Teresi, J., Holmes, D., Benenson, E. *et al.* (1993) Evaluation of primary care nursing in long-term care: attitudes, morale and satisfaction of residents and staff, *Research on Aging*, 15(4): 414–32.

Thompson, N. (1995) *Theory and Practice in Health and Social Welfare*. Buckingham: Open University Press.

Thorne, S.E. (1993) *Negotiating Health Care: the Social Context of Chronic Illness*, Newbury Park, CA: Sage.

Thorne, S. and Paterson, B. (1998) Shifting images of chronic illness, *Image: Journal of Nursing Scholarship*, 30(2): 173–8.

Thorpe, L., Davidson, P. and Janicki, M.P. (2000) *Healthy Ageing: Adults with Intellectual Disabilities – Biobehavioural Issues*. Geneva: World Health Organisation.

Thurgood, A. (1990) Seven steps to rehabilitation, *Nursing Times*, 86(25): 38–41.

Tierney, A.J. (1996) Undernutrition in elderly hospital patients: a review, *Journal of Advanced Nursing*, 23(2): 228–36.

Tilse, C. (1994) Long term marriage and long term care: 'we thought we'd be together till we died', *Australian Journal on Ageing*, 13(4): 172–4.

Titterton, M. (1992) Managing threats to welfare: the search for a new paradigm of welfare, *Journal of Social Policy*, 21(1): 1–23.

Tobin, S.S. (1996) A non-normative old age contrast: elderly parents caring for offspring with mental retardation, in V.L. Bengston (ed.) *Adulthood and Ageing: Research on Continuities and Discontinuities*. New York: Springer.

Todd, S., Shearn, J., Beyer, S. and Felce, D. (1993) Careers in caring: the changing situations of parents caring for an offspring with learning disabilities, *Irish Journal of Psychology*, 14: 130–53.

Todis, B. (1992) Nobody helps! Lack of perceived support in the lives of elderly people with developmental disabilities, in P.M. Ferguson (ed.) *Interpreting Disability: a Qualitative Reader*. New York: Teachers College Press.

Tolson, D. and McIntosh, J. (1997) Listening in the care environment: chaos or clarity for the hearing-impaired elderly person, *International Journal of Nursing Studies*, 34(3): 173–82.

Townsend, J., Frank, A.O., Fermont, D. *et al.* (1990) Terminal cancer care and patients' preference for place of death: a prospective study, *British Medical Journal*, 301: 415–27.

Travis, S.S., Duncan, H.H. and McAuley, W.J. (1996) Mall walking: an effective mental health intervention for older adults, *Journal of Psychosocial Nursing and Mental Health Services*, 34(8): 36–40.

Trieschmann, R.B. (1988) *Spinal Cord Injury: Psychological, Social and Vocational Rehabilitation*, 2nd edn. New York: Demas.

Trombly, C.A. (1995) Occupation: purposefulness and meaningfulness as therapeutic mechanisms – 1995 Eleanor Clarke Slagle Lecture, presented at the Annual Conference of the American Occupational Therapy Association, April 1995, Denver, Colorado, *American Journal of Occupational Therapy*, 49(10): 960–72.

Trydegard, G. (1998) Public long term care in Sweden: differences and similarities between home-based and institution-based care of elderly people, *Journal of Gerontological Social Work*, 29(4): 13–34.

Tuckett, D., Boulton, M., Olson, C. and Williams, A. (1985) *Meetings between Experts: an Approach to Sharing Ideas on Medical Consultations*. London: Tavistock.

Turkoski, B., Pierce, L.L., Schreck, S. *et al.* (1997) Clinical nursing judgment related to reducing the incidence of falls by elderly patients, *Rehabilitation Nursing*, 22(3): 124–30.

Turner, C. and Quine, S. (1996) Nurses' knowledge, assessment skills, experience, and confidence in toenail management of elderly people, *Geriatric Nursing: American Journal of Care for the Aging*, 17(6): 273–7.

Turner, P. (1993) Activity nursing and the changes in the quality of life of elderly patients: a semi-quantitative study, *Journal of Advanced Nursing*, 18(11): 1727–33.

Turton, P. and Faulkner, A. (1983) Carer and educator, *Journal of District Nursing*, 2: 22.

Twigg, J. (1998) Informal care of older people, in M. Bernard and J. Phillips (eds) *The Social Policy of Old Age*. London: Centre for Policy on Ageing.

Twigg, J. and Atkin, K. (1994) *Carers Perceived: Policy and Practice in Informal Care*. Buckingham: Open University Press.

Twycross, R.G. (1995) Where there is hope, there is life: a view from the hospice, in J. Keown (ed.) *Euthanasia Examined: Ethical, Clinical and Legal Perspectives*. Cambridge: Cambridge University Press.

Uitenbroek, D.G. (1996) A new public health model and ageing: the example of primary prevention by way of exercise and physical activity, *Health Care in Later Life*, 1(1): 15–27.

Usher, K. and Arthur, D. (1998) Process consent: a model for enhancing informed consent in mental health nursing, *Journal of Advanced Nursing*, 27: 692–7.

Van Gennep, A. (1995) Ageing and quality of care, *British Journal of Developmental Disabilities*, 41: 2(81): 73–8.

Van Ort, S. and Phillips, L.R. (1995) Nursing interventions to promote functional feeding, *Journal of Gerontological Nursing*, 21(10): 6–14.

Victor, C.R. (1991) *Health and Health Care in Later Life*. Buckingham: Open University Press.

Victor, C.R. (1997) *Community Care and Older People*. Cheltenham: Stanley Thorne.

Victor, C. and Higginson, I. (1994) Effectiveness of care for older people: a review, *Quality in Health Care*, 3: 210–16.

Walker, A. (1995a) Integrating the family in the mixed economy of care, in I. Allan and E. Perkins (eds) *The Future of Family Care for Older People*. London: HMSO.

Walker, A. (1995b) *Half a Century of Promises: the Failure to Realise Community Care for Older People*. London: Council and Care.

Walker, A. (1999) Older people and health services: the challenge of empowerment, in M. Purdy and M. Banks (eds) *Social Exclusion and Health*. London: Routledge.

Walker, A. and Walker, C. (1996) Older people with learning difficulties leaving institutional care: a case of double jeopardy?, *Ageing and Society*, 16: 125–50.

Walker, C. and Walker, A. (1998) *Uncertain Futures: People with Learning Difficulties and their Ageing Family Carers*. Brighton: Pavilion for Joseph Rowntree Foundation.

Walker, R.M., Schonwetter, R.S., Kramer, D.R. and Robinson, B.E. (1995) Living wills and resuscitation preferences in an elderly population, *Archives of Internal Medicine*, 155(2): 171–5.

Walley, H.M.L. (1986) *Ward Sisters' Concept of Rehabilitation*. Southampton: University of Southampton.

Walsh, P.N., Heller, T., Schupf, N. and van Schrojenstein Lantman-de Valk, H. (2000) *Healthy Ageing – Adults with Intellectual Disabilities: Women's Health Issues*. Geneva: World Health Organisation.

Warner, C. and Wexler, S. (1998) *Eight Hours a Day and Taken for Granted?* London: Princess Royal Trust for Carers.

Warner, J. (1997) Bedtime rituals of nursing home residents: a study, *Nursing Standard*, 11(20): 34–8.

Warnes, A. (1998) Divided responses to an ageing population: apocalyptic demography, ideology and rational social administration, in R. Hudson and A. Williams (eds) *Divided Europe*. London: Sage.

Waters, K.R. (1987) The role of nursing in rehabilitation care, *Science and Practice*, 5(3): 17–21.

Waters, K.R. (1991) *The Role of the Nurse in Rehabilitation of Elderly People in Hospital*. Manchester: University of Manchester.

Waters, K.R. (1996) Rehabilitation: core themes in gerontological nursing, in L. Wade and K.R. Waters (eds) *A Textbook of Gerontological Nursing: Perspectives on Practice*. London: Baillière Tindall.

Waters, K.R. and Luker, K.A. (1996) Staff perspective on the role of the nurse in rehabilitation wards for elderly people, *Journal of Clinical Nursing*, 5(2): 103–14.

Wenger, G.C. (1997) Reflections: success and disappointment – octogenarians' current and retrospective perceptions, *Health Care in Later Life*, 2(4): 213–26.

Wetle, T. (1998) Challenges and directions for gerontological research beyond 2000, *Australian Journal on Ageing*, 17(1): 107–10.

While, A. (1990) HV for the elderly, *Community Outlook*, September: 43–4.

Whitehouse, P.J., Orgogozo, J-M., Becker, R.E. *et al.* (1997) Quality-of-life assessment in dementia drug development: position paper from the International Working Group on Harmonization of Dementia Drug Guidelines, *Alzheimer Disease and Associated Disorders*, 11(3): 56–60.

Wilde, B., Larsson, G., Larsson, M. and Starrin, B. (1995) Quality of care from the elderly person's perspective: subjective importance and perceived reality, *Aging Clinical Experimental Research*, 7(2): 140–9.

Wilkes, E. (1984) Dying now, *Lancet*, 28 April: 950–2.

Wilkes, L., Bostock, E., Lovitt, L. and Dennis, G. (1996) Pressure ulcers in the older patient with a fractured neck of femur: a challenge for the nurse in the acute care setting, *Geriaction*, 14(1): 32–7.

Wilkin, D. and Hughes, B. (1986) The elderly and the health services, in C. Phillipson and A. Walker (eds) *Ageing and Social Policy: a Critical Assessment.* Aldershot: Gower.

Wilkinson, P.R., Wolfe, C.D.A., Warburton, F.G. *et al.* (1997) A long term follow up of stroke patients, *Stroke,* 28: 507–12.

Williams, B. and Grant, G. (1998) Defining 'people-centredness': making the implicit explicit, *Health and Social Care in the Community,* 6(2): 84–94.

Williams, B., Cattell, D., Greenwood, M. *et al.* (1999) Exploring 'person-centredness': user perspectives on a model of social psychiatry, *Health and Social Care in the Community,* 7(6): 475–82.

Williams, J. (1994) The rehabilitation process for older people and their carers, *Nursing Times,* 90(29): 33–4.

Williams, S.J. (2000) Chronic illness as biographical disruption or biographical disruption as chronic illness? Reflections on a core concept, *Sociology of Health and Illness,* 22(1): 40–67.

Williamson, C. (1992) *Whose Standards? Consumer and Professional Standards in Health Care.* Buckingham: Open University Press.

Williamson, J. (1988) Caring for the elderly: taking up the challenge, *Health Visitor,* 61: 17–19.

Willis, L.D. and Linwood, M.E. (1984) *Measuring the Quality of Care.* New York: Churchill Livingstone.

Willoughby, J. and Keating, N. (1991) Being in control: the process of caring for a relative with Alzheimer's disease, *Qualitative Health Research,* 1(1): 27–50.

Wills, W. and Leff, J. (1996) The Taps Project 30: quality of life for elderly mentally ill patients – a comparison of hospital and community settings, *International Journal of Geriatric Psychiatry,* 11(11): 953–63.

Wilson, H.S. (1989a) Family caregivers the experience of Alzheimer's disease, *Applied Nursing Research,* 2(1): 40–5.

Wilson, H.S. (1989b) Family caregiving for a relative with Alzheimer's dementia: coping with negative choices, *Nursing Research,* 38(2): 94–8.

Wilson, S. (1997) The transition to nursing home life: a comparison of planned and unplanned admissions, *Journal of Advanced Nursing,* 26(5): 864–71.

Wimo, A., Jönsson, B., Karlsson, G. and Winblad, B. (1998) *Health Economics of Dementia.* London: John Wiley.

Winyard, G. (1995) Improving clinical effectiveness: a coordinated approach, in M. Deighan and S. Hitch (eds) *Clinical Effectiveness from Guidelines to Cost-Effective Practice.* London: Department of Health.

Wistow, G. (1995) Aspirations and realities: community care at the crossroads, *Health and Social Care in the Community,* 3(4): 227–40.

Wistow, G. and Lewis, H. (1997) *Preventative Services for Older People: Current Approaches and Future Opportunities.* Kidlington, Oxon: Nuffield Institute for Health, Anchor Trust, Kidlington.

Woodend, A.K., Nair, R.C. and Tang, A.S. (1997) Definition of life quality from a patient versus health care professional perspective, *International Journal of Rehabilitation Research,* 20(1): 71–80.

World Health Organisation (1980) *International Classification of Impairments, Disabilities and Handicaps: a Manual of Classification Relating to the Consequence of Disease.* Geneva: World Health Organisation.

World Health Organisation (1992) *The ICD-10 Classification of Mental and Behavioural Disorders. Clinical Descriptions and Diagnostic Guidelines.* Geneva: Division of Mental Health, World Health Organisation.

World Health Organisation (1990) *Cancer Pain Relief AND Palliative Care, Technical Report Series no. 804.* Geneva: World Health Organisation.

Worth, A. (1998) Community care assessment of older people: identifying the contribution of community nurses and social workers, *Health and Social Care in the Community*, 6(5): 378–86.

Wright, L.K. (1993) *Alzheimer's Disease and Marriage.* London: Sage.

Wright, L. (1994) Alzheimers-disease afflicted spouses who remain at home: can human dialectics explain the findings, *Social Science and Medicine*, 38(8): 1037–46.

Wright, L. and Bennet, G. (1998) Telecommunication interventions for caregivers of elders with dementia, *Advances in Nursing Science*, 20(3): 76–88.

Wright, S.D., Drost, M. and Caserta, M.S. (1998) Older adults and HIV/AIDS – implications for educators, *Gerontology and Geriatrics Education*, 18(4): 3–21.

Wuest, J., Ericson, P.K. and Stern, P.N. (1994) Becoming strangers: the changing family caregiving relationship in Alzheimer's disease, *Journal of Advanced Nursing*, 20: 437–43.

Yeatts, D.E., Crow, T. and Folts, E. (1992) Service use among low-income minority elderly: strategies for overcoming barriers, *Gerontologist*, 32: 24–32.

Youdell, D., Warwick, I. and Whitty, G. (1996) *Someone to Talk to: HIV, AIDS and People over 50.* London: Health and Education Research Unit, Institute of Education, University of London.

Young, J. (1996) Caring for older people: rehabilitation and older people, *British Medical Journal*, 313(7058): 677–81.

Young, K. (1996) Health, health promotion and the elderly, *Journal of Clinical Nursing*, 5(4): 241–8.

Zarit, S.H. and Zarit, J.M. (1998) *Mental Disorders in Older Adults: Fundamentals of Assessment and Treatment.* London: Guilford Press.

Zinn, J. (1993) Inter-SMSA a variation in nursing home staffing and resident care management practices, *Journal of Applied Gerontology*, 12(2): 206–24.

Index

Page numbers in *italics* refer to tables.